State Medical Boards
and the Politics
of Public Protection

State Medical Boards
and the Politics
of Public Protection

CARL F. AMERINGER

The Johns Hopkins University Press
Baltimore and London

© 1999 The Johns Hopkins University Press
All rights reserved. Published 1999
Printed in the United States of America on acid-free paper
9 8 7 6 5 4 3 2 1

The Johns Hopkins University Press
2715 North Charles Street
Baltimore, Maryland 21218-4363
The Johns Hopkins Press Ltd., London
www.press.jhu.edu

Library of Congress Cataloging-in-Publication Data will be found
at the end of this book.
A catalog record for this book is available from the British Library.

ISBN 0-8018-5987-5

For Suzanne

CONTENTS

ACKNOWLEDGMENTS

Several organizations made information on physician discipline available to me, including the American Medical Association, the Baltimore City Medical Society, the Board of Examiners of New Jersey, the Massachusetts Board of Registration in Medicine, the Maryland Board of Physician Quality Assurance, the Federation of State Medical Boards, the Medical and Chirurgical Faculty of Maryland, and the Office of Inspector General for the Department of Health and Human Services, Boston Region. I greatly appreciate the assistance these organizations provided.

Certain individuals deserve special mention. They include Israel Weiner, John DeHoff, Michael Compton, Margaret Anzalone, and Barbara Vona of the Maryland Board of Physician Quality Assurance; Katherine Carroll of the Board of Medical Examiners of New Jersey; Margaret Burri and Steve Johnson of the Medical and Chirurgical Faculty of Maryland; James Winn of the Federation of State Medical Boards; Michael Murray and Carrie Waller of the American Medical Association; Alexander Fleming and Charles Moore of the Massachusetts Board of Registration in Medicine; Mark Yessian of the Office of Inspector General of the Department of Health and Human Services; and Bernadette Lane of the Baltimore City Medical Society. I would also like to thank Peter Dans and Henry Scagliola for their insights on current medical practice.

I am deeply indebted to my dissertation advisor, Professor J. Woodford Howard Jr., for his continuous guidance and support. Wendy Harris of the Johns Hopkins University Press managed this project to its conclusion. Mary Bleser of the University of Wisconsin–Oshkosh helped me in preparing tables and typing my manuscript. Francis Rourke, Joel Grossman, Benjamin Ginsberg, Michael Plaut, Patricia Brown, and Suzanne Fox provided comments on draft chapters. My former partners at the law firm of Niles, Barton, and Wilmer afforded me the time to devote to this effort. Barbara Francis and Debra Woodruff inspired my choice of topic. Finally, my wife, Suzanne, my children, Caroline and Katherine, and my parents, Charles and Jean, gave me their love and understanding throughout.

State Medical Boards
and the Politics
of Public Protection

The Politics of Public Protection

State medical boards, composed of doctors, lawyers, and public representatives, have evolved into the primary public institutions responsible for disciplining physicians in the United States.[1] The history of state medical boards, like that of other public agencies, is one of constant adjustment to changing political, social, and economic conditions. This is particularly true in the field of health care where the shift from professional monopoly to corporate oligopoly has disrupted long-standing ties. The ascendant role of boards as public watchdogs parallels the decline of professional authority and the rise of government and corporate bureaucracy in the health-care industry.

Whether public or private, many institutions connected with health care in the United States were, at one time, subservient to the medical profession. State medical boards were integral parts of a self-governing professional order that protected the autonomy of physicians and served their economic interests. Ostensibly created to protect the public, state boards were gatekeepers guarding entry into the medical profession rather than internal police over substandard care. They rarely disciplined physicians.[2]

Sweeping changes in the delivery and financing of health care brought discipline to prominence. New and powerful entities, including federal agencies, private insurers, and managed-care organizations, entered the health-care field in the decades following the 1960s. When the costs of providing health care skyrocketed due to expanded access and improved technology, these new entities sought to curtail spending. They restricted funds to physicians and hospitals through prospective payment and utilization review. They restructured the delivery of health care through corporate integration of medical services. Finally, they promoted competition in the medical marketplace by invoking the antitrust laws and by collecting and disseminating information on providers. These reforms permanently reconfigured the health-care landscape, shifting the balance of power from practitioners of medicine to government and corporate administrators.

Among the most significant changes were those concerning the nature of professional accountability and the role of government and corporate medicine in regulating physician behavior. Since its inception, the medical profession had claimed the right to regulate itself with a minimum of out-

I

side interference. State licensing boards were prime examples of how pro-fessions captured the police powers of state governments to perform this function. In a restructured health-care environment, government and cor-porations challenged professional self-governance on two essential grounds. First, they claimed that the profession failed to adequately police its own members. Second, they claimed that those outside the profession could do a better job of regulating the utilization and quality of medical services.[3]

Before the 1980s state medical boards rarely disciplined physicians and almost never for incompetence. In 1961 the American Medical Association (AMA) reported that "disciplinary action by both medical societies and boards of medical examiners is inadequate" and called for greater attention to "examining competence and observance of law and ethics *after* licen-sure."[4] As the recognized leader of the medical profession, the AMA's views carried great weight. Nevertheless, the profession did not always speak with one voice, particularly in the area of physician discipline. State and local (county) medical societies were functionally independent of the AMA and could formulate and pursue their own policies at the state and local levels. Because discipline was primarily a local matter, much depended on the activities of state and local medical societies. Like boards, they rarely ousted poor practitioners.

When Robert Derbyshire, a former president of the Federation of State Medical Boards, conducted his first study of disciplinary actions during the period 1963 to 1967, little had changed since the AMA report. According to Derbyshire, state medical boards disciplined about 0.06 percent of the total number of licensed physicians in any year surveyed.[5] Derbyshire conducted a follow-up study for the period 1968 to 1972 that showed a "negligible in-crease" in the number of disciplinary actions. In 1981, the first year all states reported disciplinary actions to the Federation of State Medical Boards, Derbyshire calculated that the rate of discipline had risen to 0.14 percent of all licensed physicians. Although this was an "improvement," he called this result "not impressive."[6]

Others joined Derbyshire in concluding that the medical profession was doing little to discipline doctors. Federal government studies conducted during the 1970s asserted that "disciplinary action by medical boards is almost insignificant in terms of the universe of practicing physicians."[7] A comprehensive study of medical disciplinary procedures during the 1970s by Frank Grad and Noelia Marti revealed rudimentary record keeping and "seat-of-the-pants" operations.[8] Andrew Dolan and Nicole Urban's exami-nation of medical board activities from 1960 to 1977 found that board "effec-tiveness" had improved little, if any, during that period.[9]

When medicine experienced crises in the availability and affordability of malpractice insurance in the 1970s and 1980s, some attributed the problem to the medical profession's poor performance in eliminating the small minority of physicians allegedly responsible for most of the cases.[10] Organized medicine's call for tort reform was met by efforts to upgrade physician discipline.[11] Testifying before a Senate subcommittee on tort reform measures, Otis Bowen, Secretary of Health and Human Services and a physician himself, linked the medical liability crisis, in part, to the failure of state boards and hospital peer review committees to deal with incompetent physicians.[12]

Consumer organizations recognized and began to address the problem in the 1970s. Public Citizen's Health Research Group, founded by Ralph Nader, published the first consumer's directory of local physicians in 1974. This effort encountered stiff resistance from the local medical society of Prince George's County, Maryland, where the directory was published. Because of difficulties in obtaining information on disciplinary actions, Public Citizen's first national listing was not published until 1990.[13] Released annually since then, Public Citizen's report, entitled *Questionable Doctors,* remains highly critical of medical boards for not doing enough to protect the public.

Media criticism of board performance became particularly intense during the 1980s. The *Washington Post* decried "the secrecy, lack of public accountability and poor coordination between state boards, the AMA and other medical monitors" (1 Sept. 1985). The *New York Times* acknowledged complaints that "no one was policing the medical profession adequately" (2 Sept. 1985) and its headlines scolded: "Doctors Who Get Away with Killing and Maiming Must Be Stopped" (2 Feb. 1986). Certain commentary referred to state medical boards as "a public health vacuum" (*Nation's Health,* Apr. 1990). Several embarrassing exposés blamed the medical establishment for board inaction. Articles in the *Washington Post* noted the inherent conflict between "goals of protecting a doctor's rights and protecting the public" (10 and 11 Jan. 1988). Stories in the *Boston Globe* stressed the political activities of state medical societies in thwarting board initiatives (11 Dec. 1989).

Responding to these and other failures, government and private enterprise developed alternative mechanisms for controlling physician behavior. These included government-sponsored peer review, utilization review, risk management, and quality assurance programs. Although government-sponsored peer review organizations (PROs) often engaged professional associations to review medical practice, the others did not. Utilization review organizations, for instance, usually employed nurses and other medical personnel to screen treatment decisions. Administrators of hospitals and other entities used risk management and quality assurance programs to monitor physician performance externally.

These devices allowed managers and administrators to regulate the physician-patient relationship on the basis of financial performance as well as professional competence. Whether these and other means of controlling physician behavior actually rid the medical profession of poorly performing physicians was doubtful. Little evidence existed to show that they did. PROs, for instance, rarely sanctioned physicians for substandard care. In 1992 PROs made only fourteen recommendations nationwide to exclude physicians from participation in Medicare and Medicaid programs.[14] Moreover, PROs rarely shared information about quality-of-care programs with state medical boards.[15] The same was generally true of risk management and quality assurance programs in hospitals and managed-care organizations, despite state laws that required these entities to report poor performance to state boards.[16]

No one doubted that government and corporations regulated physicians more than in the past. The question was whether added scrutiny actually improved public protection or served the economic interests of the new players, just as self-regulation had improved the financial lot of physicians. Business, at least, seemed more interested in containing costs or in making profits than in protecting the public from poor practitioners.[17] While scientific methods of assessing physician performance, such as outcomes research, clinical guidelines, and other data-intensive efforts, promised to improve overall quality from an institutional perspective, the public also required protection from physicians who were guilty of incompetence or unprofessional conduct.[18] When it came to physician discipline, boards were about the only game in town.[19]

Change across the Boards

Deepening hostility toward self-regulation suggested that state medical boards faced extinction unless they improved their performance. Most boards responded in three general ways. First, boards changed their focus from licensure to discipline. Second, boards developed the bureaucratic machinery to handle difficult and complex cases on their own and without the help of organized medicine. Third, boards became an information resource for government, consumers, and health-care entities such as hospitals and managed-care plans.

In a self-regulating system, boards were gatekeepers, nothing more.

Having the authority of the state behind them, they set the criteria and decided who could practice medicine and who could not. As protectors of the public and of the integrity of the medical profession, they went after "quacks," "charlatans," and other "unorthodox" providers of medical care. Few boards looked inward toward the medical profession itself. Subscribing to a professional ethic, they relied on normative pressures to control the behavior of licensed physicians. There was no perceived need to develop the institutional capacity required for disciplining physicians on a grand scale.

Following government intervention, the medical field became a public arena in which formal rules and procedures prevailed. Normative pressures were no longer sufficient to force compliance with ethical and practice standards. This meant that boards, to remain viable, had to change their focus from guarding the gates to minding the store. Although state medical societies often opposed enforcement efforts, most boards changed their focus from licensure to discipline in the 1970s and 1980s. According to data generated by the Federation of State Medical Boards, reported actions against physicians resulting in loss or restriction of licenses increased almost eightfold from the early 1980s to the mid-1990s (see table 2.1 and figure 2.1 later in this book).

This did not alleviate concerns about the quality of board actions and their consequences for the public and the profession.[20] According to Public Citizen, discipline remained a problem in 1996. "Though it has been vastly improved during the past 15 years," the consumer organization asserted, "the nation's system for protecting the public from medical incompetence and malfeasance is still far from adequate."[21] Public Citizen estimated that boards should discipline at least 1 percent of doctors each year or 6,233, a number substantially greater than the 2,675 "serious" disciplinary actions it counted in 1996.[22]

Boards also recast their agenda by embracing issues of public concern, such as unprofessional conduct and substandard care. In a self-regulating environment, cases came to boards from law enforcement agencies or from medical societies with much of the work already completed. Boards were endpoints in a system designed to secure the power of the medical profession. Although consumer groups and the media clamored for boards to take on high-profile and difficult cases, most boards had neither the inclination nor the wherewithal to pursue them. Several obstacles stood in their way, including the medical profession itself. As Derbyshire noted, "the curtain of silence is all too prevalent. Many doctors are aware of incompetence or wrongdoing on the part of their colleagues, yet refuse to report them to the authorities."[23] Board members were volunteers, without legal training or time for lengthy proceedings. Boards had no trained staff to undertake detailed investigations or to review voluminous medical records. They were principally small-scale operations, not complex bureaucratic organizations.

Initial efforts by boards to pursue incompetence and unprofessional conduct signaled a transformation in professional attitudes and the status of boards as regulatory bodies. During the period 1963 to 1967, boards prosecuted a total of seven cases of incompetence; from 1986 to 1996, boards prosecuted 1,677 such cases.[24] Although Public Citizen noted that "only a minority of physicians were given disciplinary actions which stopped them, even temporarily from practicing,"[25] the implications were clear. Boards had gained the funding and hired the staff needed to initiate investigations and to prosecute cases on their own. Some board members even expressed concern that bureaucratic management might override professional judgment.[26]

Finally, boards became a clearinghouse for information concerning poor practitioners. Board parochialism long had been a barrier to information sharing and publication. The Federation of State Medical Boards, founded in 1912, seemed a likely candidate for coordinating board activities. Although the federation had collected and disseminated information on formal disciplinary actions since 1915, its data were inconsistent and incomplete until advances in computer technology provided a cost-effective means for collecting and processing large amounts of information.[27] The first year the federation obtained uniform reporting from all member boards was 1984. In 1985 the federation issued its first annual summary of reported disciplinary actions. By then, most states required health-care entities and insurance carriers to report hospital restrictions and malpractice claims. Boards collected these and other data, took action if appropriate, and advised the federation.

Although of value to boards and other government agencies in detecting offenders, federation data were not for public consumption. Consumers had to contact their boards directly or obtain Public Citizen's listing for their state of residence. Even then, consumers could find out only if a physician's license had been revoked or restricted in some fashion. Boards rarely informed the public of physicians under investigation, and until 1997 no board released information on malpractice actions or hospital discipline.[28]

Despite advances in disciplinary performance and information dispersal, boards faced an uncertain future. Managed care rapidly changed the focus of regulatory initiatives. By 1995 more than 80 percent of physicians were affiliated in some way with an organization that practiced case management and used a combination of financial incentives and utilization review to contain costs.[29] Patients switched health plans, not doctors. Under the circumstances, government and consumer groups moved toward developing measures of performance, such as quality report cards, that assessed an entire organization. Boards were rarely, if ever, mentioned in these efforts.[30]

Nevertheless, the conduct of individual physicians remained central to patient care and was becoming harder to evaluate, particularly in instances in which physicians' loyalties were divided among patients, institutional providers, and managed-care plans.[31] Financial concerns affected medical judgment in the past, but money was now front and center.[32] Physicians needed help in navigating the corporate minefield. Organized medicine claimed that business and professional concerns could be reconciled without altering long-standing relations between physicians and their patients.[33] State medical boards subscribed to this viewpoint but seemed unsure of their future role. Whether boards stayed on the sidelines or became central figures in this debate could shape the outcome. Much depended on the scope of conflict among professional, government, corporate, and consumer interests.

The Scope of Conflict

The political scientist E. E. Schattschneider asserted that "the outcome of all conflict is determined by the *scope* of its contagion."[34] In other words, the number of participants and the nature of their involvement decide the result of any controversy. Politics, he said, was about controlling conflict in ways that benefited the individuals or groups involved. Those that succeeded in managing the scope of conflict would prevail. Powerful interests would seek to keep disputes private so as to control the number of participants and the terms of the debate. Weaker interests would appeal to public authority for redress of private grievances. According to Schattschneider, these "conflicting tendencies toward the privatization and socialization of conflict" framed all political struggles.[35] Was this also true of political struggles among the medical profession, government, business, and consumer interests in the health-care arena? Did the privatization and socialization of conflict play a central role in physician discipline?

Schattschneider's thesis explains the dynamic role of boards in public protection. In the nineteenth century, physicians faced extensive competition from those within and outside the medical profession. Under siege, professional leaders appealed to state governments to limit the supply of physicians and to regulate the activities of nonphysician practitioners. Boards were a result of medicine's campaign for economic protection.[36] When physicians became the dominant power in health care over the course of the next several decades, boards operated as the profession's gatekeepers by excluding untrained and unqualified practitioners through licensure and other legal means. Using boards to limit the scope of conflict within the medical field was a strategic move, and one that Schattschneider clearly foresaw. Just as licensing restrictions governed the allocation of tasks within hospitals and the behavior of workers, they also provided a "normative shield" against government regulation and private suits for malpractice.[37]

Government intervention in the medical field expanded the scope of conflict and reshaped existing alliances. According to Schattschneider, "the trends toward the privatization and socialization of conflict have been disguised as tendencies toward the centralization or decentralization, localization or nationalization of politics."[38] Resolving conflicts on the local level were a means of restricting their scale. So long as boards remained minor operations without the staff and resources to tackle tough cases, local medical societies and community hospitals handled complaints by patients against their physicians. This changed in the 1970s when lawsuits against professional societies and hospitals for violations of antitrust laws made private enforcement risky. The crisis in medical malpractice insurance and media exposés of bad doctors also gave the impression that self-discipline was nonexistent. The combined effect was to expand conflict from the local to the state and national levels and from the private to the public domain. Boards now had to confront a growing caseload.

Once in the public spotlight, boards came under the scrutiny of federal and state governments that had invested heavily in health care under the Medicare and Medicaid programs. Federal and state authorities expected a return from their investment and became anxious when the costs of health care grew out of control. Blaming physicians in part for the problem, the federal government reviewed the performance of doctors and prosecuted them for health-care fraud and abuse. State governments looked to boards for assistance in policing the medical community. When not forthcoming, several states seized control of board operations and functions, often requiring boards to use and share investigative and other resources under the direction of a central agency. According to the Office of Inspector General for the Department of Health and Human Services, the number of boards under state agency control increased from sixteen in 1969 to thirty-one in 1986.[39] States also expanded board size and composition to include nonphysician members. Most boards today have at least one or two nonphysician members; thirty years ago there were almost none.

Schattschneider's thesis anticipated these events. Government's entry into the health-care field altered the balance of power. "The function of democracy," Schattschneider argued, "has been to provide the public with a second power system, an alternative power system, which can be used to counterbalance the economic power."[40] In the 1970s the countervailing power to government in health care was the medical profession. As Paul Starr clearly demonstrated, professional authority extended well beyond the clinical realm, engulfing markets and institutions.[41] Boards represented an extension of professional control. For years they were free to protect the interests of the medical profession while acting as agents of state government. Now that government itself had entered the fray, boards were caught in the middle of a power struggle that involved organized medicine on one side and the public interest on the other.

The economist Paul Feldstein offered an additional perspective on the widening conflict in health politics. Applying economic theory, Feldstein asserted that changes in health policy occur after groups having a diffuse cost develop a concentrated interest. According to Feldstein, physicians prevailed until the 1960s because they were the only group with a significant stake in health economics. State medical boards failed to monitor physicians because organized medicine opposed government regulation of private practice. Increasing costs of health care adversely affected government budgets and corporate profits during the 1970s and 1980s. Feldstein concluded that the predominant interests of government and corporations in controlling costs led to measures that weakened the political influence of organized medicine.[42]

Concentrated interests of government, business, and consumer groups widened the scope of conflict over physician discipline in the 1970s. As Schattschneider recognized, everything changed once conflict became political. The shift in focus from licensure to discipline, the development of a bureaucracy to handle difficult and complex cases, and the collection and dissemination of information on physicians' backgrounds took place after new stakeholders emerged to weaken physicians' power. Seizing control of the regulatory apparatus was part of government and corporate strategy, just as it had been for organized medicine.

With the passage of legislation establishing health maintenance organizations (HMOs) in the early 1970s, the federal government moved toward a market competition model in the medical field. According to Starr, "the socialized medicine of one era had become the corporate reform of the next."[43] Despite their many changes over the last fifteen years, boards were part of the old power structure. Subscribing to Schattschneider's belief that "the function of institutions is to channel conflict," corporate providers of health care fashioned their own organizations, such as the National Committee for Quality Assurance, with ties to federal and state governments.[44] Dismissing the role of boards as regulators of health quality, HMOs maintained that state insurance departments, though ill-equipped, were more appropriate for monitoring their activities.[45]

The failure of federal efforts to reform health care in the 1990s meant that powerful entities in the private sector would determine the shape of the delivery system. Now it was the medical profession, as the weaker party, that sought to expand the scope of conflict by invoking the public interest to achieve legislative action. The recent spate of laws banning gag clauses in HMO contracts, promoting due process protection for physicians fearing termination from health plans, and mandating certain benefits, such as minimum lengths of maternity stays in hospitals, are prime examples.

Boards did their part to cultivate an image that appealed to a wider audience. By disseminating information about physicians, boards became players in an emerging network that stressed consumer choice as key to cost control. By emphasizing the accountability of physicians to their patients for incompetence and misconduct, boards filled a gap in the system for regulating the quality of health care. Seeking to stem the tide of corporate medicine, physicians embraced board initiatives to counterbalance external control.

A Preview of Things to Come

The political maelstrom surrounding state medical boards reflected the widening scope of conflict in health policy during the last thirty years. A number of other institutions with strong ties to the medical profession, including hospitals, medical schools, and insurance companies, also struggled to accommodate both public and private concerns. Their leaders shifted strategies and reformed their organizations during the transition from a professional monopoly to a corporate oligopoly. Like boards, they encountered resistance from professional, government, business, and consumer groups.

What set boards apart was their role in making public policy. How boards exercised this function reflected the degree of professional control over the health-care system. Chapter 1 describes the formation of state medical boards and their efforts to protect and maintain professional authority. Seeking to keep disputes private, boards rarely disciplined licensees. That was the job of state medical societies, medical staff of hospitals, and other credentialing bodies. As public agencies, boards restricted the supply of physicians through licensure and prosecuted nonphysicians for the unauthorized practice of medicine. The lines were clearly drawn to contain the scale of conflict.

Rapid changes in technology, coupled with increased demand for medical services following World War II, exposed weaknesses in the professional order. Medical education and training in schools and hospitals were insufficient to ensure competence over a doctor's career. Efforts to address a shortage of practitioners caused many physicians to practice beyond their means and hospitals to rely on foreign-trained physicians, many of whom performed poorly on state board examinations, to fill residency positions.

Seeking to contain the growing conflict over poor performance, state and local medical societies formed grievance committees in the 1950s and 1960s to resolve disputes among physicians and their patients. Grievance committees gave consumers an outlet for their complaints while preserving professional values and customs through case mediation. State medical boards relied on grievance committees for resources and expertise, just as in later years many depended on peer review committees and impaired physicians programs of state and local medical societies for investigation and rehabilitation of offenders. By using grievance committees to monitor the direction and flow of cases, organized medicine maintained control of the disciplinary process.

Chapter 2 relates how the playing field shifted in the 1970s. Efforts to control costs stymied organized medicine but presented new opportunities for its rivals. The professional order declined, and a new order, characterized by regulation of the medical profession through government and corporate bureaucracy, began to emerge. Federally sponsored peer review organizations and other government agencies sought to supplement or replace traditional mechanisms for maintaining physician competence and ethical standards. State governments centralized board operations, added consumer members to board panels, and restricted the role of state medical societies in the selection of physician members. These efforts undercut organized medicine but did not substantially increase the number of disciplinary actions taken. Just as organized medicine hindered board initiatives, so too did state government. State budgets, rules, and regulations constrained board powers, reducing their flexibility. Board parochialism persisted under central agencies in several states.

Chapter 3 describes how the Federation of State Medical Boards sought to curtail government takeover of board operations. As early as 1956, the federation promoted a "model" state board that was independent of other branches of state government.[46] By the late 1980s the federation's version had reconciled differences among professional and bureaucratic forms of organization. The new model superimposed a collegial body, composed mainly of physicians, on top of a central bureaucracy, composed mainly of professional bureaucrats.[47] Similar to a private corporation, the former managed the organization while the latter handled the day-to-day affairs. Physician control of the entire operation through a board of directors was key. Under the federation's guidance, many boards became self-funded entities, hired their own staffs, and established their own networks for exchanging information. In the wake of these developments, actions against physicians resulting in loss or restriction of licenses increased substantially in the 1980s. Cases involving substandard care, incompetence, or negligence achieved priority.

Although the effect of these changes was to channel conflict in directions more amendable to the medical profession, tensions between boards and state medical societies increased when boards recast the agenda in the 1970s and 1980s to accommodate government and consumer interests. For several years, these former allies waged battles over issues such as physician drug abuse, sexual misconduct, and physician incompetence. Chapter 4 relates these various battles.

Stressing confidentiality, self-reporting, and rehabilitation, state medical societies formed impaired physicians programs (IPPs) in the 1970s when the problem of physician drug abuse gained national attention. Because most IPPs refused to share names of impaired physicians with state boards, government officials and the press raised concerns about the role of IPPs in protecting the public. The matter received widespread attention, particularly in New Jersey, where a government investigation, court litigation, and media publicity expanded the scope of the conflict.

Public recognition of physician sexual misconduct occurred in the late 1980s. In Massachusetts, attempts by the state board to prosecute certain high-profile cases created a backlash in the medical community. For the next several years, the state board was at the center of a controversy that pitted professional societies against consumer groups. The case study of sexual misconduct in Massachusetts demonstrates that powerful private interests use government to contain conflict, just as weaker interests appeal to government to expand it.

Chapter 4 also examines the problem of physician incompetence. This issue, more than any other, captured the growing controversy among public and professional interests. Although physicians claimed the right to determine the competence of fellow practitioners, professional associations lacked hard evidence showing that they were successful in controlling offenders, particularly in the 1970s and 1980s when crises in medical malpractice insurance gained prominence. As Schattschneider would have predicted, state and local medical societies formed peer review committees in the early 1970s to privatize the conflict. Few besides Maryland's medical society succeeded in conducting formal peer review as an agent of the state medical board. Because of its appeal to organized medicine, the AMA officially endorsed the "Maryland Model" in 1991.[48] Public and private partnerships between boards and state medical societies reconciled the demands of government administrators for quality control and those of medical practitioners for substantive authority, just as they did in the case of federal peer review organizations.

Attempts to moderate differences between boards and medical societies gained momentum in the 1990s as managed care became the principal tool for undermining professional dominance. Chapter 5 describes how organized medicine appealed to consumers, courts, and government to restore the balance between cost and quality in the provision of medical services. For their part, boards sought to regulate utilization review activities of HMOs. These efforts led to court confrontations that would eventually determine whether boards participated in the emerging power structure.

Chapter 6 reviews the transformation of state medical boards and examines their place in the new corporate order. Corporate integration of the health-care industry has profound implications for the regulation of the medical profession. The revolution that is reshaping the delivery of medical services is also recasting the regulatory landscape. It already has changed professional, managerial, and legal practices. Physicians have altered their behavior under capitated payment systems that encourage underutilization of medical services. Managers have adopted continuous quality improvement and other techniques that stress teamwork and enhance the roles of nonphysician providers. Lawyers have pursued enterprise liability and other legal theories to recover money damages against health-care facilities.

Underlying these changes is a diffusion of political, social, and economic power. The decline of the professional order and the fragmentation of the medical community has fostered reliance on state medical boards and courts to police professional misconduct. Boards have seized the initiative in responding to the interests of consumers and government officials. But while old problems persist, new ones emerge. Profit-maximizing behavior of HMOs will test physicians' allegiance to individual patients, and disciplinary rules and professional ethics governing doctor-patient relations will often conflict with corporate norms of behavior.

CHAPTER ONE

The Professional Order

Many observers have envisioned the struggle for power in American society largely as a confrontation between two major power systems, government and business.[1] In health care, the primary confrontation was between the federal government and organized medicine. The medical profession's highly publicized campaign against "socialized medicine" during the administrations of Presidents Franklin Roosevelt and Harry Truman epitomized this struggle. Until the enactment of the Medicare and Medicaid programs in 1965, organized medicine prevailed, not only against the federal government but also against other forms of competition in the private sector.[2]

A key part of organized medicine's success was the formation of a professional order that kept conflict private and its competition in check. This order consisted of institutions that physicians established or promoted to serve their interests—professional associations, medical boards, medical schools, and hospitals; the laws that protected them; and the political, social, and economic ties that bound them. These institutions held sway for most of the twentieth century. During medicine's Golden Age, from about 1945 to 1965, physicians reached the pinnacle of autonomy, free from outside interference and dominant over all others in the medical field.

Each component of the professional order had a role to play. Professional associations were the primary political institutions of organized medicine. Arranged hierarchically, they included the AMA and state and local (county) medical societies. These entities formulated policy and developed strategy for achieving the goals and objectives of physicians at the national, state, and local levels. State medical boards, the public arm of the state medical societies, were the profession's gatekeepers. They licensed the qualified, banished the unqualified, and shielded the profession from external review. Medical schools and hospitals were the educational and clinical components of the professional order. Physicians used these institutions to ensure competence, control supply, and reduce competition.

The formation, development, and evolution of state medical boards closely track the rise to power and domination of organized medicine in the health-care industry from the late 1800s to the 1960s. Although boards had the authority to discipline offenders under the public law, few actually did, relying instead on state and local medical societies, hospitals, and their own informal procedures to control misconduct.[3] These approaches kept disputes among physicians and their patients private, so as not to tarnish the idealized image of the medical practitioner as a person worthy of the public's confidence and trust.[4] Boards went public only to attack chiropractors and other competitors who threatened medicine's dominance in the private sector.

The medical profession would eventually pay a price for its avoidance of formal disciplinary action. When public criticism of the medical profession mounted in the 1950s and 1960s, boards and professional associations had little to show for their past efforts. Even the AMA, on completion of its eight-year study of medical discipline in 1961, expressed dissatisfaction with the lack of centralized reporting, so successful had the profession been in channeling conflict through local institutions.[5] Changing public perceptions of medicine and of professions in general created the need for enhanced oversight and accountability. Medicine's leaders were well aware that if the profession did not act, government would.[6]

Competition in the Medical Marketplace

The triumph of professionalism in the early twentieth century secured a place for physicians in a newly industrialized nation. Reforms in education and licensing restricted the supply of physicians and instilled professional values in future generations. Changes in hospital management gave physicians authority over all clinical matters. Reorganization of the AMA cemented relations with state and local medical societies and increased membership in associations. These and other efforts helped physicians achieve complete autonomy and eliminate competition.

The medical profession did not obtain its lofty status overnight. Unbridled competition plagued the medical profession for much of the nineteenth century. During the Jacksonian period, legislatures repealed laws enacted in many states delegating licensure authority to medical societies. Lacking controls on physician supply, the number of physicians practicing in the United States exceeded existing needs. Few made a good living in the healing arts.[7] States licensed prospective candidates whether they graduated from a state-chartered medical school or they passed a test administered by a state medical society following a period of apprenticeship.[8] Aggravating the situation further, medical sects or cults proliferated. First on the scene were the Thompsonians, who subscribed to the "natural" remedies of botanic medicine. Other groups succeeded them, including eclectics, homeopaths, osteopaths, Christian Scientists, and chiropractors. Most formed societies and established schools that rivaled conventional or allopathic medicine.[9] Bitter disputes between sectarians and regular practitioners ensued. Physicians attacked sectarians claiming they were "quacks" or "charlatans" who were incompetent to treat human ailments.[10] Sectarians responded, accusing physicians "of seeking a monopoly for their own benefit."[11]

Although physicians sought to regulate competition and impose uniform standards, economic, social, and technological conditions were not conducive to success in the early and middle 1800s.[12] Because of the immature state of science and technology, medical care took place in patients' homes where physicians could best apply their clinical experience and judgment in diagnosis and treatment. Any existing hospitals were charitable facilities that administered to the poor. Physicians with paying clients had little need for hospitals or for other physicians. Consequently, medical societies could not control physicians' behavior in the absence of licensure and other institutional mechanisms. As Starr has noted, "The orientation of the profession, in short, was *competitive* rather than *corporate*."[13]

Reacquiring the authority to license became a paramount concern of professional leaders. Circumstances changed enough near the end of the nineteenth century to make this possible. Advances in science and technology, coupled with the industrialization and urbanization of American society, encouraged specialization and interdependence among physicians and their economic rivals. Collaboration among physicians and sectarians in the private sector led to some interesting bedfellows in the public sector. Because physicians lacked the political punch to secure the passage of licensing laws on their own, they needed the help of "irregular" practitioners.[14] These collaborative efforts eventually bore fruit. In 1875 Texas established the first state board of medical examiners.[15] By 1900 most states had enacted laws calling for the licensure of physicians.[16]

Despite ethical prohibitions against association with unorthodox providers, allopaths served with homeopaths and eclectics on several state licensing boards. Chiropractors, osteopaths, and optometrists secured independent board status.[17] Nevertheless, the medical profession's goal was a single licensing board for each state composed exclusively of physicians.[18] With the assimilation of homeopaths and eclectics into the dominant allopathic regime, the profession's goal became a reality.[19] In state medical boards, organized medicine gained the public authority to attack its rivals and, at the same time, to keep conflicts affecting the public private.

Medical societies in each state handled problems involving untrained practitioners and sectarians differently, but most followed a similar pattern. In Maryland, for example, the state legislature in 1798 incorporated a "soci-

ety of physicians" known as the Medical and Chirurgical Faculty (Med Chi)
and granted it licensing powers.[20] An exception permitting graduates of the
University of Maryland College of Medicine to practice medicine without
a license appeared after 1812.[21] In 1838 Thompsonians successfully challenged Med Chi's exclusive authority and secured the passage of a law giving every Maryland citizen the right "to charge and receive compensation"
for medical services.[22] An early Med Chi historian characterized the situation as follows: "At [one] stroke . . . free enterprise in medical practice re-
turned to its colonial status. The Thompsonian craze subsided in a short
time, as similar products of mass psychology have done before and since;
but the effect of the lawmakers' unintelligent surrender to it remained in
force and was not remedied until half a century later."[23]

Although Thompsonianism faded in Maryland as elsewhere, other rivals to allopathic medicine materialized. Consequently, Med Chi did not
obtain licensing authority again until 1892.[24] The 1892 act established two
separate boards of medical examiners in Maryland, one representing Med
Chi and the other representing the Homeopathic Society. Under the act,
each society appointed board members free from outside interference.
Maryland maintained separate boards until the demise of the Homeopathic
Society in 1957.[25]

Court decisions supported the grant of public authority by state governments to the medical profession. The first challenge to medical licensing
laws occurred in West Virginia following the conviction of Frank Dent, an
eclectic physician, under a 1882 law for practicing without a valid license.[26]
Claiming the law violated the Fourteenth Amendment's due process clause,
Dent asked the U.S. Supreme Court to find the law unconstitutional.
Holding against Dent, the Court acknowledged West Virginia's right to
provide for the general welfare by requiring that practitioners of medicine
possess the "necessary qualifications of learning and skill."[27] Although the
Court had previously invoked "substantive due process" to protect "individual rights over special privilege conferred by the states,"[28] professions,
particularly medicine, were different. Writing for a unanimous Court, Justice Field stated that "few professions require more careful preparation by
one who seeks to enter it than that of medicine." The "subtle and mysteri-
ous" nature of medical practice, he continued, assured that "comparatively
few can judge" a physician's qualifications.[29]

The Supreme Court also accepted the view that licensure was in the
public interest. State courts agreed. According to one state court, the purpose for the passage of legislation establishing medical boards was to protect the public "from the consequences of ignorance and incapacity in the

practice of medicine and surgery."[30] State medical boards were eager to sustain this view. In 1923 Maryland's board reported to the state medical society that "at the time of its adoption the country was overrun with poorly trained and self-appointed medical men, and *it was to protect the public* that Licensing Boards were established, the idea being that the Boards would license only such persons as gave assurance of being qualified to practice healing" (italics added).[31]

Dent settled the matter of a state's power to license professions in the public interest, but certain issues remained unresolved. One such issue concerned whether a state could delegate licensing authority to a private entity, as Maryland had done in the case of Med Chi. The Supreme Court did not reach this issue in *Dent* because West Virginia vested licensing powers in its State Health Board. Courts in Maryland, Indiana, California, and Iowa rebuffed these challenges, finding that delegations were permissible.[32] The Supreme Court would not entertain constitutional challenges to licensing board composition again until the 1970s.[33]

Although founders of state medical boards went out of their way to justify medical licensure, they seemed far less concerned about medical discipline. Among the initial reasons for revocation of a license were "habitual drunkenness, criminal abortion, conviction of crime involving moral turpitude or unprofessional or dishonorable conduct."[34] Early medical society bylaws added "ethical violations" to this short list.[35] There was no ground for "technical incompetence." If medical societies in the nineteenth century expelled physicians, it was not for incompetence. Rather, it was because they practiced in an "unconventional" manner or competed unfairly through advertising.[36]

The decision to exclude "technical incompetence" as a ground for revocation in early licensing laws was entirely consistent with English precedent. Seeking to explain this possible shortcoming in British law, A. M. Carr-Saunders and P. A. Wilson offered two theories.[37] First, they surmised that because medicine was an inexact science, the treatment of disease required "good judgment." In occupations such as ship navigation or mine inspection, by contrast, where the "observance of routine" was essential to avoid disaster, the public demanded mere technical competence. Although technical competence was also important for doctors and lawyers, they argued that overemphasis on "rule-of-thumb methods" would undermine initiative. Second, they noted that the practice of medicine encompassed many different approaches. Boards composed of physicians, they suggested, might engage in "heresy-hunting" should they have the power to enforce certain standards.

Recent emphasis on incompetence as a basis for disciplining physicians highlights changes in the medical field. If Carr-Saunders and Wilson were correct in their assessment of early disciplinary grounds, then the fundamental perception of medicine as an inexact science, incompatible with routine or standardized procedures, has changed. Growing consensus concerning the diagnosis, treatment, and prevention of disease partially explains this phenomenon. The remainder of the explanation lies in the bureaucratization of medical practice.

Determining Competence through Licensure and Credentialing

Another plausible explanation for the failure to include "technical competence" as a ground for medical discipline is reliance on credentialing to assure proper performance. Credentialing is the principal mechanism that professions use to ensure competency, control supply, and reduce competition. In the medical profession, doctors obtain credentials through medical education and training, licensing, hospital privileging, and specialty board certification. The evolution of public and private credentialing bodies was closely tied to medicine's success. Organized medicine secured power by controlling organizations that produced new physicians and structured medical practice. In the case of institutional credentialing, organized medicine procured laws and regulations that vested decision-making authority in private entities under its control. In the case of individual credentialing, where state medical boards preexisted educational reform, it captured control of board operations.

Reducing the number of medical schools that produced poorly trained physicians crowned the AMA's agenda following its political reorganization in 1901. Starting in 1906, the Council on Medical Education (CME), an AMA-sponsored organization, began a series of inspection tours designed to standardize medical training and admissions policies. Based on what it found on its first inspection tour, the CME devised a rating system and classified medical schools according to the quality of their programs and their requirements for admission and graduation. The CME targeted for closure all schools that did not achieve a 50 percent rating.[38]

During the CME's second tour of inspection in 1909–10, Abraham Flexner issued his now famous report for the Carnegie Foundation criticizing medical education in the United States.[39] Although the Flexner Report helped publicize serious deficiencies in medical school education, the CME had done much of the spade work and was well on its way to correcting the situation. Many medical schools were not able to remain open under the

CME's watchful eye. In 1904 the United States had 162 medical schools, more than all other countries combined. By the end of 1918 only eighty-five schools survived, the product of several closures, mergers, and other consolidations. The CME's success in reducing the number of medical schools hinged on the passage of laws making licensure contingent on graduation from a board-approved school. Because state medical boards did not have sufficient resources to compile an approved list of medical schools on their own, many relied on the CME to do it for them. In 1912 two different organizations representing boards in connection with their licensing activities merged to form the Federation of State Medical Boards. Soon after its formation, the federation sanctioned the CME's rating system for medical schools.[40]

There were now two private organizations, the CME and the Federation of State Medical Boards, that set public standards for physician licensure. This arrangement would serve as a precedent for organizing future relationships between public and private entities where professional interests were concerned. In 1927 the journal of the AMA proudly announced that

> since the investigation and classification of medical schools began, licensing boards in gradually increasing numbers have secured legislation authorizing them to refuse to examine graduates of low grade medical schools. By 1920 the diplomas issued by such schools were scarcely worth the paper they were printed on in all but a few states. Since 1920, indeed, only three states, Arkansas, Connecticut, and Florida, continue to provide wide open doors for the licensing of poorly qualified doctors.[41]

While the CME reviewed medical schools and internship training, the American College of Surgeons (ACS), another private entity, appraised the nation's hospitals. Based on its first survey conducted in 1919, the ACS approved only 89 of the 692 hospitals that it reviewed. Hospitals seeking approval after 1919 steadily conformed to ACS standards for medical staffing and patient care. By 1950 the ACS had approved 3,290 hospitals.[42]

In 1951 the Joint Commission on Hospital Accreditation (JCAH), organized under the auspices of the AMA and other voluntary associations, succeeded the ACS. JCAH surveys were entirely voluntary and confidential and, like ACS surveys, focused on medical staff and patient care issues. When the federal government came on the scene in 1965, physicians successfully wrote into federal legislation that JCAH-approved hospitals were "deemed" to be in compliance with Medicare standards for participation. States that licensed hospitals also adopted JCAH accreditation requirements.[43]

Besides setting a precedent for hospital accreditation, the American College of Surgeons was the prototypical specialty board. The transition to specialty practice in the early decades of the twentieth century was anything but smooth. Generalists harbored deep resentment for specialists who achieved higher income and prestige. The Annual Report of the Council of Medical Education to the AMA House of Delegates in 1921 noted that changes in medical practice had created "two classes of medical men, the generalist and the specialist," and that medical faculties often excluded the former. Revealing a distinct bias in favor of generalists, the CME stated that the "narrow specialist may do a great deal of artificial and unnecessary work and if uncontrolled may be a menace to his patients and to sound medical practice." The CME called upon state medical boards to regulate specialty care.[44]

Specialists would have none of this. Oliver Garceau, a professor of government, conducted a demographic survey of organized medicine for the years 1923–38 which showed that urban specialists had captured control of key positions within the AMA and state medical societies.[45] Generalists, as the CME report attests, also held power. The result for specialty licensure must have been a deadlock. Neither side was willing to forego the privilege to perform medical work in any particular area.[46] As occurred elsewhere, a private settlement resolved this dispute.

Because a general license to practice medicine set no restrictions on specialization, hospital privileges were the principal means for determining competence. Licensed physicians seeking to treat patients in a hospital setting had to become members of the medical staff and obtain clinical privileges. Gaining medical staff membership required that physicians meet certain criteria, not the least of which included medical school graduation, followed by internship and licensure. Specialty board certification might also be a criterion for medical staff membership. Before delineating clinical privileges, credentialing committees of hospitals considered specialty background, including board certification.[47]

Beyond the hospital setting, no private entity was responsible for ascertaining the technical competence of physicians on a continuing basis in their private practice. Because of their licensing and disciplinary powers, state medical boards were the most likely candidates. Boards, however, lacked legal grounds to discipline physicians for incompetence before 1965.[48] Allowing boards to discipline doctors for incompetence would have required the formulation and enforcement of uniform standards. Disputes among generalists and specialists indicated that political infighting discouraged such efforts. Physicians emphasized either medicine's art form or its scientific basis to suit their interests. Medicine as art furthered professional autonomy. Medicine as science thwarted competition. State medical boards were gatekeepers, nothing more. Their jobs were to limit access to the medical profession and to police its boundaries. For boards, the scientific basis of medicine was a sword.

Medical Discipline before World War II

As with licensing, medical discipline was largely a family affair. State medical boards complemented other components of the professional order to achieve a climate conducive to professional domination and control of the health-care industry. Boards were endpoints in an informal disciplinary process that sought to curtail governmental and corporate intrusions on professional autonomy.

Although organized medicine often wielded boards as clubs to deter ethical misconduct, formal discipline in the form of a suspended or revoked license was rare. Despite the lack of formal discipline, physicians, for the most part, were kept in line through a network of institutions operating at the local level. This highly decentralized approach to physician discipline contained the scope of conflict, much as Schattschneider envisioned. Boards were not supposed to discipline offenders except for the most serious offenses.[49] An AMA survey in the 1950s of state medical boards and medical societies stated that, "almost without exception, discipline is a local matter, and since county societies handle discipline, the states have little or no knowledge of what is being done."[50] The role of boards was to support professional interests at the local level. This was the essence of self-governance. Because boards were public entities operating at the state level, any regulatory activities directed toward physicians threatened the professional order.

In 1847 the AMA adopted a Code of Ethics based on the work of Thomas Percival, an English physician. The Code of Ethics and subsequent revisions appearing in 1903, 1912, 1949, and 1957 supported sanctions against physicians for fee splitting, contract practice, advertising, and other forms of "unfair" competition.[51] Not until the early 1900s was judicial machinery in place to interpret and enforce ethical principles.[52] State societies adopted the AMA's Code of Ethics and enforced its provisions through their judicial councils.[53] By 1920 medical boards in several states had included disciplinary grounds for fee splitting and contract practice.[54] If a particular ethical principle was not listed among the grounds for discipline, boards could still charge physicians with "unprofessional conduct" or "professional misconduct."[55]

Studies of the medical profession's rise to power during the twentieth century argued that medical ethics were "political and organizational tools."[56] Writing in 1942, physician Frank Riggall acknowledged that "codes of ethics are used for the benefit of doctors and not patients."[57] Their principal goal was to encourage and maintain professional autonomy. For instance, the prohibition on fee splitting supported professional autonomy by preventing hospitals from paying physicians to join their medical staffs.[58] The prohibition on contract practice discouraged physicians from forming or joining medical cooperatives that promoted group practice, prepayment, preventive medicine, and consumer participation. Because such activities threatened traditional forms of payment and increased the potential for third-party involvement, some medical societies expelled participating physicians. Celebrated expulsions involved founders of clinics in Los Angeles, Elk City (Oklahoma), Milwaukee, and Chicago.[59] In 1938 the Justice Department initiated and eventually convicted the AMA under the Sherman Antitrust Act for conspiracy to prevent the operation of the Group Health Association, a Washington, D.C., cooperative.[60]

Despite the availability of sanctions for unprofessional conduct, actual prosecutions were few and far between.[61] In 1932 the Judicial Council of the AMA acknowledged the reluctance of physicians to prosecute colleagues who violated medical ethics. As the council reported:

> Few individuals feel it their personal responsibility to prosecute a breach of ethics that affects them personally but little but which may affect the profession of medicine in a major degree. The institution of charges by an individual in such cases of general concern might very probably in many instances amount to professional suicide, and seldom does any individual desire to place himself on his own initiative in the position of prosecutor for the benefit of the profession as a whole and bring on himself the unfriendliness and antagonism of colleagues often in influential positions.[62]

To ease the stigma on an individual physician, the Judicial Council recommended to the House of Delegates that local medical societies establish a "system of medical jurisprudence" similar to that in "society as a whole." By this, the Judicial Council meant an independent body that would bring an indictment and an independent prosecutor who would represent the medical profession. Although some local societies gave these recommendations serious consideration, they were largely ignored.[63]

When it came to professional discipline, the growth in power and prestige of organized medicine discouraged aberrant behavior. Because a physician's economic survival often depended on acceptance by the local fraternity, medical societies rarely had to revoke a license or expel one of their members to prevent future misconduct.[64] Besides coverage for malpractice, society membership brought patient referrals and consultations, hospital access, and professional appointments.[65] The importance of these benefits to individual physicians reflected their growing interdependence. Societal changes arising from industrialization, urbanization, and immigration required major adjustments to the way physicians had practiced medicine in the nineteenth century. Specialization was the principal means of coping with these changes. Most specialists practiced in urban settings with access to hospital and research facilities. Because of the importance of referrals by colleagues, the practice of medicine evolved from one that was "client dependent" to one that was "colleague dependent."[66]

Hospital affiliation was critical to a physician's success. During organized medicine's formative years, hospitals "moved from the periphery to the center of medical education and medical practice."[67] Just as revenues from patient care fueled hospital expansion, so physicians gained a powerful voice in hospital administration. Unlike the situation in Europe, where a salaried staff supervised patient care, private physicians maintained control after their patients entered a hospital. This "peculiar" arrangement prevented hospitals from achieving the degree of integration more typical of formal organizations. Physicians sought a centralized administration to coordinate hospital operations, but their resistance to hierarchical authority separated clinical from administrative control.[68] Hospital administrators and physicians shared authority at the top of distinct theaters of operation.

Because physicians required the "sponsorship" of an elite group of community practitioners to secure hospital privileges, entrenched practitioners had the power to exclude those deemed unacceptable.[69] A potential source of exclusion was lack of membership in a local medical society. In 1934 the House of Delegates of the AMA linked hospital access to society membership by passing the Mundt Resolution, which conditioned hospital accreditation for internship training on the affiliation of the medical staff with a local medical society.[70]

Physicians ostracized from medical societies had few avenues of relief. Until the 1970s, practitioners could not invoke federal antitrust law for wrongful denial of society membership because courts had held that the practice of medicine did not affect interstate commerce.[71] Those seeking hospital privileges who had not been initiated into the local fraternity might not get them. The first court case providing relief against a private hospital for denial of staff privileges was not until 1963.[72]

Court rules and doctrines codified physician autonomy while deferring to the profession's methods of internal governance. The locality rule encouraged professional unity in malpractice cases. The corporate practice of medicine doctrine, based on the failure of corporations to satisfy conditions for personal licensure, helped secure professional autonomy by preserving fee-for-service practice.[73] So did the refusal of courts to hold hospitals vicariously liable for the conduct of their medical staffs.[74] Underlying these decisions were professional interests that courts expressed as public policy concerns, among them lay control over professional judgment, commercial exploitation of medical practice, and the potential division of physician loyalty between patient and employer.[75]

The driving force behind physician self-regulation before World War II was professional autonomy. Professional politics, ethics, and accompanying laws promoted internal cohesion and discouraged government, corporations, insurance companies, and even patients from interfering in professional matters. As long as political, social, and economic forces sustained an atmosphere where professions could flourish, physician discipline was self-contained. Doctors who misbehaved were rarely punished through formal means. Fear of ostracism was often sufficient to discourage aberrant behavior. Private controls sufficed.

Policing the Boundaries of the Medical Profession

At common law, anyone could practice medicine. The only real checks on the competence of practitioners were lawsuits for malpractice. Although states had the right to prevent incompetents from practicing medicine, they rarely exercised this prerogative. Caveat emptor—"let the buyer beware"— was the controlling principle. By enacting legislation that established medical boards in the late 1800s, states recognized that medical practice required "special knowledge" and that patients lacked the ability to judge qualifications. The right to practice medicine was now "subordinate to the police power of the State to protect and preserve the public health."[76]

State officials delegated to the medical profession the power to decide what the practice of medicine was and who had the right to practice it. Because of their education and training, physicians claimed that they were the only ones competent to practice medicine. Determining where the boundaries lay between the authorized and unauthorized practice of medicine occupied the attention of organized medicine during its formative years. It was in the profession's interests to extend the boundary lines of medical practice as far as possible. State medical boards played a key role in this effort.

Early laws defined the "practice of medicine" broadly and made few exceptions for nonphysicians. Georgia defined practice of medicine to include "the diagnosis or treatment of disease, defects, or injuries of human beings, or the suggestion, recommendation, or prescription of any form of treatment for the . . . relief, or cure of any . . . ailment."[77] The Georgia law excluded dentists and veterinarians from its provisions. Maryland's definition encompassed anyone "who shall operate on, profess to heal, prescribe for, or otherwise treat any physical or mental ailment."[78] Dentists and "druggists" were the only groups excluded from the requirements of the Maryland law. In the absence of a specific statutory provision, Pennsylvania courts found that practice of medicine "covers and embraces everything that by common understanding is included in the term healing art."[79] Similar definitions prevailed in other states, the principal distinguishing features being physicians' ability to prescribe drugs and perform surgery.[80]

Confronted with these broad jurisdictional claims, competitors, particularly osteopaths and chiropractors, sought protective legislation. In 1941 the Nebraska Medical Association conducted a survey of medical practice acts in thirty-seven states.[81] The survey revealed that osteopaths and chiropractors had secured at least limited licenses to treat disorders of the human body in most states. Osteopaths fared better than chiropractors. In about half the states surveyed, osteopaths could engage in the general practice of medicine, including administering drugs and performing surgery, if they satisfied general licensure requirements for allopathic physicians. Otherwise, osteopaths could obtain a limited license to practice osteopathic medicine.[82] Chiropractors had no right to practice medicine.[83] Three states, Louisiana, Mississippi, and Texas, denied them the right to practice at all.[84]

Organized medicine publicly attacked chiropractors and other groups, branding them "cultists" and claiming that they lacked sufficient education and training. In 1919 the CME declared that "the medical profession is justified in objecting to the various cults, not because of their peculiar system of practicing but because of their serious lack of education and the fact that they are seeking the right to practice as physicians without meeting the same educational standards with which physicians have to comply."[85] According to the secretary of California's Board of Medical Examiners, chiropractic schools were deficient in their entrance requirements, course of study, and laboratory equipment. He charged that such schools trained graduates to "defy the law and denounce all regulations except by a chiropractic board."[86] In the view of physicians who were delegates to the annual convention of the Federation of State Medical Boards in 1928, cultists were the "enemy."[87]

Despite intense efforts by physicians to denounce them, chiropractors made inroads among America's middle and lower classes.[88] Medical boards pursued several options to stem the "chiropractic wave sweeping over the country."[89] One option was to prosecute chiropractors for violating state medical practice acts.[90] From 1906 to 1936, there were reportedly more than fifteen thousand prosecutions.[91] The most active state boards were in New Jersey, New York, California, Kentucky, and Ohio. New Jersey's board alone prosecuted over four hundred cases in 1928.[92] Yet chiropractors remained openly defiant of state medical boards. Many used the title *physician,* a designation customarily restricted to practitioners of medicine.[93] The Federated Chiropractors of America adopted the slogan "Go to jail for chiropractic."[94]

Physicians often doubted that criminal sanctions were netting results. Aggressive enforcement of medical practice acts in Ohio and California produced a sympathetic backlash.[95] At the federation's convention in 1928, some delegates advocated "self-improvement and public instruction" over criminal prosecution. One of the convention's speakers, Ray Lyman Wilbur, United States Secretary of the Interior, referred to "irregular practitioners" as "simply sparks that fly off the anvil." The Surgeon General of the United States also warned against too much enforcement, stating that "the profession might be compared to an army which had erected a very high brick wall directly in front of it but had left its rear and both flanks exposed."[96]

Reassessing its approach, organized medicine took steps to deny licenses to chiropractors. Several state medical societies pressed legislatures to adopt basic science laws for the purpose of testing all candidates for licensure in the healing arts. In those states that adopted basic science laws, chiropractic boards could not issue licenses unless candidates first passed the requisite test. Wisconsin was the first state to enact such a law in 1925. At least twenty-three more states followed suit during the next thirty-five years.[97] By establishing separate "nonprofessional" boards, advocates of basic science laws added another layer onto the already rigorous licensing requirements for doctors. If the idea was to bar chiropractors from licensure, the attempt apparently backfired. According to Derbyshire, the "high failure rate" among physicians and the loss of reciprocity between licensing boards was a high price to pay for excluding "a few chiropractors, many of whom can pass the examination, anyway."[98]

The reliance that organized medicine placed on state boards to deter chiropractors from practicing medicine diminished with advancements in science and technology and the institutionalization of the medical field. So long as the provision of health services was privately controlled, physicians had the upper hand. Without proper credentials, individual providers operated on the periphery of the health-care system, forever banished from medical facilities and patient referral networks. Membership in a medical society, with all its benefits, was closed to nonphysicians. Hospital medical staffs denied privileges to osteopaths, chiropractors, chiropodists, and others. Medical ethics forbade physicians from associating with "unscientific practitioners."[99]

By midcentury, physicians dominated the medical field. The period from about 1945 to 1965 was known as the "Golden Age" of medicine. According to Eliot Freidson, a professor of medical sociology, this was a period when medicine "was at a historically unprecedented peak of prestige, prosperity, and political and cultural influence—perhaps as autonomous as a profession could be."[100] Several groups, including opticians, masseurs, midwives, optometrists, and physical therapists, secured the right to practice, but they did so within carefully defined areas.[101] In most instances, the division of labor benefited physicians who used subordinate groups to expand their authority.[102] Where physicians failed to reconcile their differences with a competitor, as in the case of chiropractors, they persisted in their efforts to eliminate them.[103]

The dominance that physicians achieved came at a price. In Freidson's view, part of that price was the need for the medical profession to "control deviant performance and to regulate itself in general."[104] The preoccupation of organized medicine with protecting its turf from outsiders undermined such efforts. Physicians labeled nonphysicians "incompetent," not their colleagues. Yet competence was a question that physicians would have to face, particularly since their licenses gave them such broad jurisdictional powers. Once physicians conquered or, at least, diminished the threat of medical cults, they had to face their own detractors. The situation was not unlike that of the end of the Cold War.

Storm Clouds on the Horizon

Despite medicine's acknowledged success in dominating the healthcare field, its public image suffered in the years following World War II. According to historian John Burnham, "the rare public doubters of the medical profession in the late 1940's and early 1950's gradually increased in number."[105] Early critics of physicians focused on excessive fees and indifference to the personal concerns of patients. Eventually even the technical performance of physicians became suspect as lawsuits for medical malpractice increased in number, particularly in the 1970s. By then, the prestige of the profession had declined to the point where government and corporate insurers could safely intervene in medical decision making. What transpired to bring this about?

While there is no simple answer, state medical boards shared in the blame. Their attacks on chiropractors and their efforts to limit the number of licensed physicians won them few friends outside the medical community. At times, their tactics were heavy-handed. Just as boards waged war against chiropractors, so they also used oral interviews to exclude some qualified candidates for medical licensure. According to one leading physician, "Some individuals were of the wrong sex. Some were of the wrong race. Others were of the wrong religion. Still others were planning to compete with members of the board or their friends. The interview was a convenient way to refuse a license to anyone who was considered undesirable."[106]

But more than anything else, it was lack of disciplinary action against poor practitioners that rallied public opinion against the medical profession. Physicians were naturally reluctant to discipline their colleagues. Because clinical practice was case-specific, physicians relied on their own instincts, based on personal experience. Criticizing fellow colleagues was bad form since mistakes were inevitable. Making such concerns public was particularly inappropriate because it might encourage a lawsuit for malpractice.[107] According to Freidson, good practitioners simply avoided poor ones. The mechanism of personal, or "colleague-group" boycott, was the preferred course of action, not disciplinary sanctions.[108]

The failure of physicians to adequately police their ranks led to claims that a "conspiracy of silence" flourished in the medical community. Among the first to popularize this notion was Philip Wylie, author of the book *Generation of Vipers* and a series of articles in *Redbook* magazine in 1952. Wylie castigated physicians for neglecting their public duties and for branding as traitors those physicians who reported their harmful colleagues: "Whether or not doctors have the sole legal right to be judges of themselves is not exactly open to question; by and large, they do have it. Whether or not they should have so much authority, is a different question. And part of its answer depends upon how well they 'police' themselves. It is my contention that they do a wretched job of it."[109]

In often graphic detail, Wylie related instances in which physicians had misdiagnosed illnesses, performed unnecessary surgeries, and botched simple operations. Wylie drew attention to the fact that little was ever done about these bad apples. He was not alone. Several other critics wrote books and articles in the 1950s that reproached physicians for failing to take disciplinary action.[110]

Concerned about the inhospitable climate, professional associations responded by forming grievance committees in the early 1950s to hear complaints from patients against their physicians. By 1961 over eleven hundred such committees coexisted with state and local disciplinary bodies.[111] Physicians who were reluctant to discipline their fellow colleagues had fewer qualms about mediating complaints. Originally established to resolve relatively minor disputes over issues such as excessive fees, many grievance committees of local medical societies gradually expanded their jurisdiction to include cases of serious physician misconduct. Committee members often investigated complaints alleging substandard care or unethical practice. If complaints called for disciplinary action, committee members referred them to state medical boards or judicial councils of state medical societies. Organized medicine still viewed state medical boards as institutions of last resort.

By way of example, the Professional Relations Committee of the Baltimore City Medical Society was central to Maryland's disciplinary framework. It screened and resolved a large number of complaints alleging physician misconduct. Table 1.1 shows the number and distribution of cases that the Baltimore City Medical Society handled from 1955 to 1973.

Specific referral patterns emerged among entities involved in disciplining physicians in Maryland. Med Chi, the state medical society, often referred cases to the Professional Relations Committee of Baltimore City and committees of other local societies for investigation and mediation. In most instances, the local society resolved the matter. If not, Med Chi reviewed the case on appeal and, in certain instances, referred it to the state board with a recommendation for disciplinary action. The local society could also bypass Med Chi and refer a case directly to the state board.[112] Table 1.2 reflects the number and distribution of cases involved in Maryland's case referral network during the 1960s. Table 1.3 shows the actual number of disciplinary actions Maryland's board compiled in those same years.

The number of case mediations reported in table 1.1 contrasts sharply with the number of disciplinary actions reflected in table 1.3. From 1961 to 1971, the Baltimore City Medical Society alone mediated over 750 complaints, while the state board disciplined a total of only sixty-eight doctors. One apparent explanation for the disparity is that disciplinary actions were the culmination of a formal legal process sometimes pursued following unsuccessful case mediation. To physicians, discipline represented a breakdown in the educational system. Those punished were beyond hope; public officials had to deal with them.

Grievance committees and state medical boards were not in conflict. Each supported the other. Lacking resources to investigate and screen cases, boards relied on state and local societies to do much of the spade work. Lacking authority to subpoena records or discipline offenders, state and local societies used the threat of board sanctions to induce physicians to

TABLE 1.1
Complaints against Physicians Mediated by Baltimore City
Medical Society, 1955–1973

Year	Fees	Treatment	Ethics	Other	Total
1955–57	16	9	6	15	46
1958	22	12	11	10	55
1959	15	2	11	6	34
1960	30	6	16	4	56
1961	18	5	13	7	43
1962	16	3	18	13	50
1963	13	12	9	14	48
1964	15	6	6	25	52
1965	17	11	4	25	57
1966	18	2	7	13	40
1967	35	6	1	29	71
1968	43	14	11	15	83
1969	35	11	29	2	77
1970	45	25	37	0	107
1971	71	20	33	0	124
1972	68	34	30	0	132
1973	59	32	63	0	154

Source: Data from Baltimore City Medical Society.

Note: Fees refers to complaints about physician fees such as overcharging, double billing, or charging for services not performed. *Treatment* refers to complaints about improper or inadequate medical care, including misprescribing of drugs, sexual contact with a patient, or malpractice. *Ethics* refers to complaints about ethical misconduct, including advertising, unnecessary surgery, and fee splitting. *Other* refers to complaints that did not fall into any of the categories listed. Some cases covered more than one category. If a case involved *treatment*, I elected that category over the other two. If a case involved *ethics* and *fees* only, I chose *ethics.*

comply with their procedures. In certain instances, grievance committees even persuaded physicians to surrender their licenses in order to avert disciplinary action.[113]

Combining the activities of state and local grievance committees with those of state boards paints a different picture from that depicted in public accounts. For all their reluctance to sanction colleagues, physicians actively investigated allegations of incompetence and unprofessional conduct when adjusting patient grievances. As shown in table 1.1, physicians resolved a substantial number of these complaints. Lack of formal discipline and standardized reporting obscured their efforts.

The AMA Calls for a New Approach to Disciplining Physicians

Not all professional leaders, particularly those at the national level, believed that old approaches to disciplining physicians sufficed.[114] Some advocated greater involvement by state medical boards in the disciplinary process and more centralized reporting of data on physician misconduct. Speaking before the Federation of State Medical Boards in 1961, Raymond McKeown, a member of the AMA's Medical Disciplinary Committee, remarked, "There cannot be and there will not be progress if each county medical society acts independently of its neighbors, if the state association is not aware of what its components have done, if the AMA is not permitted to act as a clearinghouse for all state and county societies. This is even more true with state boards."[115]

TABLE I.2

Distribution of Cases among Med Chi and Component Medical Societies, 1961–1971 (Based on Cases Referred)

Year	Baltimore City M.S.	Other Local M.S.	State M.S. (Med Chi)	State Board*
1961	39	37	7	
1962	46	42	10	
1963	48	31	6	
1964	46	53	11	2
1965	53	67	25	1
1966	37	63	7	6
1967	59	75	52	13
1968	83	83	46	12
1969	77	126	66	12
1970	97	163	62	14
1971	122	196	32	10

Source: Data from Mediation Committee, "Annual Reports to the House of Delegates," *Maryland State Medical Journal* (July 1962): 423; (July 1963): 359; (Aug. 1964): 93–94; (Aug. 1965): 85–86; (July 1966): 102–3; (May 1967): 67–68; (July 1968): 82–84; (July 1969): 100–101; (June 1970): 70–71; (July 1971): 84–85; (August 1972): 64–65.

Note: Reports are based on information from previous calendar years. The Mediation Committee began reporting cases in 1961. In September 1972 the Mediation Committee changed its name to the Physician/Patient Relations Committee. There are no published reports of case mediations after 1971.

*Information on referrals to state board is not available before 1964.

TABLE 1.3

Disciplinary Actions by Maryland State Board, 1961–1971

Year	Revocations	Suspensions	Reprimands	Other	Total
1961	3	0	0	4	7
1962	2	1	0	4	7
1963	1	0	0	2	3
1964	3	0	0	1	4
1965	1	0	1	5	7
1966	0	0	5	4	9
1967	2	1	4	2	9
1968	1	0	0	5	6
1969	0	0	0	2	2
1970	0	0	7	2	9
1971	1	1	2	1	5
Total	14	3	19	32	68

Source: Data from Annual Reports and Minutes of Maryland board for available years.

Note: Reports reflect revocations, suspensions, reprimands, and various other types of procedures, including revocations with stay (probations) and license denials. Obtaining an accurate picture of the actual number of physicians that state boards prosecuted before the mid-1980s is difficult, because much relevant information is incomplete or nonexistent. One must exercise caution when comparing results in earlier years with those in later years, because the number of licensed physicians had increased and disciplinary bodies had secured more flexible sanctioning authority.

McKeown and his colleagues began collecting information on state medical boards and state medical societies for the AMA in 1953. They did not complete their work until 1961, at which time they published their findings in a report to the AMA's Board of Trustees (the AMA Report). The lengthy period of investigation was due, in part, to the committee's difficulties in obtaining hard data. Despite several requests for information, only thirty-seven boards and thirty-eight societies eventually responded to its questionnaire. Frustration with the lack of responses and details received was evident in the committee's published findings. This experience alone convinced committee members that "discipline is either something of secondary importance or something not to be discussed."[116]

In spite of incomplete information, committee members pieced together a picture of board and state medical society operations. They found "wide variation" in the size of boards, ranging anywhere from five to fifteen members, and a small number of osteopaths, chiropractors, and chiropodists on some boards (20). Most state medical societies played an active role in choosing board members by recommending nominees to the governor for appointment (32). Rather than selecting board members for their "judicial" skills, the committee discovered that societies chose board members "on the basis of teaching or scientific accomplishments—or as an honor to a respected practitioner" (54).

The committee reported that relationships among boards and medical societies were "informal but cooperative" (22). For the most part, there was free exchange of information between these entities because their members served in dual capacities, had common secretaries, or shared the same office space (23, 54). Few states adopted formal rules to handle disciplinary matters, despite the promulgation of the Model State Administrative Procedure Act in 1946. Only two states, California and Oregon, prepared annual reports of disciplinary actions (21). Funding for board operations was "inadequate" and showed great disparity, ranging anywhere from a few thousand to over four hundred thousand dollars (23, 54).

Among the grounds for disciplining physicians, nine were common to medical practice acts in thirty states. These grounds included drug addiction, unprofessional conduct, fraud in connection with examination or obtaining a license, alcoholism, advertising, illegal abortions, conviction of an offense involving moral turpitude, and mental incompetence. More than eighty other disciplinary offenses were scattered throughout various state laws. Disciplinary grounds contained in medical society bylaws exhibited a corresponding lack of uniformity (31–32, 41–43).

The committee found that state boards revoked the licenses of sixty-eight physicians in 1960 and that state societies expelled or suspended sixteen physicians in 1960 (App. 3a, 3b). Considering that there were over 250,000 physicians in the United States in 1960, committee members concluded that "disciplinary action by both medical societies and boards of medical examiners is inadequate" (46). They called upon state boards to "seriously consider the advisability and necessity of making discipline their primary responsibility" (68). Among the committee's recommendations for improving discipline were standardization of medical practice acts and rules of procedure, annual reporting of disciplinary activities to a central repository, and retention of legal counsel to minimize error in board proceedings (67–69).

Few state medical boards followed the committee's advice. As reflected in table 1.4, total disciplinary actions for all boards combined remained roughly the same for each year during the 1960s. According to Derbyshire, these numbers showed that boards disciplined about 0.06 percent of the total number of licensed physicians in any given year.[117] Almost half of all disciplinary actions concerned violations of narcotics laws, and most of the

TABLE I.4

Disciplinary Actions by State Medical Boards, 1960–1968

Year	Revocations	Suspensions	Other	Total
1960	70	—	—	554
1961	102	—	—	604
1962	72	66	329	467
1963	75	43	283	401
1964	83	42	282	407
1966	69	45	465	579
1968	64	60	397	521

Source: Data from Judicial Council, "Medical Disciplinary Reports," JAMA 190 (1964): 1077; JAMA 194 (1965): 124; JAMA 202 (1967): 165; JAMA 210 (1969): 1092–93. — = no reported actions.

remaining cases consisted of actions for unethical conduct or for mental illness. Seven cases (or less than 1 percent) involved "gross malpractice." Although Derbyshire observed that "professional incompetence" was "one of the most vexing problems facing the state boards," he noted that it was rarely listed as a ground for discipline.[118]

Some boards were more successful than others in disciplining poor practitioners. For example, California's board took fifty-nine disciplinary actions in 1963, eighty-five in 1964, seventy in 1966, and sixty-seven in 1968.[119] Board members in California attributed their success to the board's proactive role in spotting problem physicians by monitoring court records, mental hospital admissions, and narcotics prescriptions. Physician William Quinn, a member of California's board, agreed with the AMA's medical disciplinary committee that efforts of boards "have largely ceased with the discharge of the licensing function." Quinn noted that to improve discipline, California's board increased its budget through licensing fees and hired fifteen investigators.[120]

Despite corrective action by a few states, professional leaders knew that more was required to avert government intervention in the disciplinary process.[121] In his monthly message to the medical profession in 1958, AMA president David Allman beseeched physicians to act more responsibly: "Any reluctance to reprimand an erring colleague does irreparable harm to our profession. Any use of a whitewash brush to sweep dirt under the rug imperils our disciplinary system. Any compromise with personal moral convictions damages the very character which makes a man or a woman a good doctor."[122] At the annual meeting of the Federation of State Medical Boards in 1962, speaker after speaker extolled the delegates to action. In the words of one, "The criticism continues and grows. The stature of the profession is being eroded—piecemeal." If physicians are not more vigilant, he warned, "a state or federal legislature [might] seize the initiative."[123]

Boards were in a precarious position. Their mission was changing because of evidence that medical education and training were inadequate to ensure competent performance over a doctor's career. The public expected boards to take a more pronounced role in disciplining physicians, but they were unable to do so because of existing constraints. Boards depended on professional associations and state governments for resources and guidance. Neither was particularly forthcoming in the 1960s. Unless physicians' attitudes changed and government and organized medicine committed more resources to the effort, as in California, formal disciplinary actions would remain constant for the foreseeable future. Altering the character of physician discipline would require more than intermittent public outrage and a few critical studies. Several forces would have to interact over time to disrupt the medical field and transform boards as institutions.

Conclusion

State medical boards were key factors in organized medicine's rise to power in the early twentieth century. At a time when competition among practitioners was keen, boards provided legal authority to restrict the supply of physicians and to define the scope of medical practice. Once its power was secure, organized medicine used boards as shields against government and corporate intervention in its internal affairs. Boards adopted ethical prohibitions on fee splitting, contract practice, advertising, and other forms of "unfair" competition to support the profession's monopoly of health care. To gain a foothold in the health-care industry, federal officials and corporate providers would have to overcome the rules that boards and professional associations forged to govern medical practice.

In all other respects, boards were weak participants. They fulfilled a public function, but what occurred behind the scenes was more important. Other organizations—hospitals, professional associations, and private credentialing bodies—assumed prominence in licensing and disciplining physicians. For example, the Council on Medical Education took the lead in approving medical schools and hospitals for internship training. Boards piggybacked the CME's efforts when they licensed graduates of approved schools. The same was true of discipline. Because most cases involved criminal offenses, unethical conduct, or mental illness, those that reached state medical boards usually originated in the courts or the professional associations. Before the 1960s, few boards even considered regulating professional incompetence after licensure.

Those critical of board efforts often overlooked the highly decentralized nature of the disciplinary process. State medical boards posed a threat to local interests if they disciplined large numbers of physicians for incompetence. Such an undertaking required adequate staff to review complaints, obtain and evaluate medical records, and interview witnesses. It also compelled board members to hire attorneys to advise them on legal matters and prosecute cases. Boards would remain small-scale operations, with little staff and few resources of their own, so long as organized medicine confined the scope of conflict to the private sector. Discerning the problem, those on the AMA's Medical Disciplinary Committee offered this advice: "Any planning to initiate a more effective system of discipline must recognize the fact that disciplinary functions are highly localized, and any attempt to assume aggressive leadership in effecting changes in the present system is likely to meet with [substantial] obstacles."[124]

The formation of grievance committees in the early 1950s reflected physicians' avowed preference for private mediation over public discipline. Grievance committees were tools for containing the scope of conflict. They kept certain basic principles intact: professional judgment, local control, and self-regulation. Adhering to these basic principles helped maintain professional autonomy just as it preserved the discrete and insular relationship between physician and patient. With physician as mediator, personal grievances could be adjusted without public consequences. Patients retained their privacy and physicians their integrity. Contrast this with formal discipline that entailed public ridicule for offenders and the medical profession at large.

What was missing from this process was the public. There was little protection for the public if physicians were allowed to adjust grievances in private to avoid public disclosure. Although national leaders like McKeown warned that boards needed more money, resources, and legal authority to do the job, local and state medical societies failed to support these efforts.[125] According to McKeown and his coauthors of the AMA Report, organized medicine had the "personnel, funds, and channels of communication" to make the needed changes, but "lack of forceful leadership" meant that state medical boards would continue to discipline only the worst offenders.[126]

To maintain the status quo, organized medicine kept state medical boards subordinate to state medical societies. Societies in many states controlled the selection of board members, housed their operations, and managed their staff. This approach was compatible with the long-standing strategy of medicine to capture government agencies by making them dependent on private organizations for resources and expertise. So long as boards lacked the ability to handle large numbers of complex cases, local interests prevailed. As Schattschneider predicted, conflict was contained. Professional associations were successful until state governments began to consolidate board operations in the 1960s.

CHAPTER TWO

The Decline of the Professional Order

Before the 1970s the medical field was relatively stable because of the medical profession's dominant position. Despite continuing skirmishes with chiropractors, physicians had eliminated most of their competition. The profession set the rules for its members, hospitals and other health-care facilities, and allied health professionals. Although many individuals had insurance coverage, insurance companies exercised little control, if any, over the selection of physicians and the conduct of medical practice.[1] Federal and state governments rarely interfered. Just as many private-sector firms induced government to formulate rules that benefited their operations, the medical profession used government to benefit physicians. Medical boards were primary examples.

For almost a century, boards followed the lead of state and local medical societies. Their mission was to control competition within medicine, which they did primarily through licensing. Growing public discontent with the medical profession led to the AMA's recommendation in 1961 that boards reevaluate their performance. Despite genuine efforts by some boards to improve, there was little overall gain in numbers of physicians disciplined during the 1960s, as the data in table 1.4 indicate. There were two main reasons for this. The first was boards' dependence on private professional associations to frame and direct their activities. So long as organized medicine dominated the health-care industry, it resisted formal sanctions against physicians for unprofessional conduct or incompetence. These were areas where the profession traditionally asserted almost exclusive jurisdiction. The second reason, related to the first, was inadequate organization and resources. Because regulation of physician behavior was localized, privatized, and decentralized, state boards never developed the capacity for managing a complex and growing caseload.

Revolutionary changes in the health-care industry over the next thirty years altered the context for medical discipline. A restructured system for delivering health care affected traditional roles of key players, including physicians, hospitals, patients, insurers, and government regulators. Professional accountability increased once institutional providers of medical services faced the need for cost containment and quality control. Efforts of government to regulate physician behavior gained priority in a competitive market. Once state medical boards adapted to this new environment, the number of disciplinary actions taken against licensed physicians substantially increased. Figure 2.1 depicts the rise in disciplinary activity starting about 1984.[2] Table 2.1 shows that increased disciplinary activity outpaced the number of new physicians entering the medical profession.

Starting in the 1970s, federal and state governments, courts, consumers, and the press began to widen the scope of conflict in the health-care field and to weaken the ability of organized medicine to govern itself. Promoting a market competition model to control costs, the federal government opened the medical field to antitrust regulation. Antitrust actions against professional associations and medical staff of hospitals undermined local means of regulating physician behavior, as did crises in the availability and affordability of medical malpractice insurance in the 1970s and 1980s. Attributing the malpractice crises in part to poor self-regulation, states scrutinized board operations, altered the composition of board panels, and changed the means of selecting board members. States also required courts and insurance carriers to report malpractice cases to medical boards. Finally, consumer groups and the media pressed boards to discipline physicians for a variety of offenses, including drug abuse, sexual misconduct, and incompetence.

By the late 1980s the transition from self-regulation to government regulation, from primarily private to primarily public enforcement, and from decentralized to centralized controls was virtually complete. Although some of the increase in disciplinary actions in the mid-1980s, as shown in figure 2.1, was probably due to enhanced reporting and data-collection activities of the Federation of State Medical Boards, sustained efforts by boards to discipline offenders signaled the development of complex organizations that were responsive to consumer needs.

The Big Picture

Federal enactment of the Medicare and Medicaid programs in 1965 sowed the seeds of instability in the medical field. Government subsidization of health care occurred earlier in the form of funding for the construction of public health facilities, but it never before involved direct payment for care. Although organized medicine opposed national health insurance, it eventually supported more limited types of coverage for the poor and aged. The profession's central interest was in preserving the physician-patient relationship. So long as third parties did not interfere in medical decision making, physicians were not opposed to expanded forms of insurance coverage.[3]

Professional support for Medicare and Medicaid stemmed from the

FIGURE 2.1

Disciplinary actions by state medical boards, 1969–1995.

Source: Data for the years 1969–78 from Derbyshire, "Medical Self-regulation," 197. Data for the years 1981–95 from the Federation of State Medical Boards.

Note: Total actions include license revocations, suspension, surrenders, probations, restrictions, denials, and reinstatements. Total number of actions for 1969–78 was 3,623.

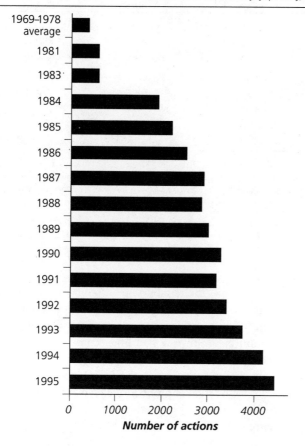

retrospective method of payment for health services that Congress originally adopted. Federal and state governments reimbursed providers of medical services for "reasonable costs" incurred in rendering care. Because there were few restrictions on payment for services performed, providers had little incentive to control costs. Several other developments also encouraged overspending, such as new technology, expanded liability on the part of physicians and hospitals for medical injury, and a professional and societal ethic that called for physicians to provide patients with the best care avail-

TABLE 2.1
Disciplinary Actions per Thousand Nonfederal Patient-Care
Physicians, 1969–1995

Year	Actions per 1,000 Physicians	Year	Actions per 1,000 Physicians
1969–78	avg 1.21/yr	1989	6.27
1981	1.53	1990	6.71
1983	1.39	1991	6.31*
1984	4.48	1992	6.56
1985	5.12	1993	7.06
1986	5.69	1994	7.74
1987	6.30	1995	7.79
1988	6.07*		

Source: Data for the years 1969–78 from Derbyshire, "Medical Self-regulation," 197. Data for the years 1981–95 from Federation of State Medical Boards. For the number of nonfederal patient care physicians, Lillian Randolph et al., *Physician Characteristics and Distribution in the U.S.* (Chicago: American Medical Association, 1996–97), 35.

Note: Actions includes license revocations, suspensions, surrenders, probations, restrictions, denials, or reinstatements.

*Estimated.

able. Under the circumstances, the reimbursement policy was a potential financial disaster. From 1967 to 1983, Medicare spending rose from $3 billion to over $37 billion.[4] Cost-containment measures were inevitable.

Federal subsidization of health care had other consequences as well, chief among them the growth of commercial enterprise. Before the involvement of the federal government, there were relatively few commercial investors in medical-care facilities. Nonprofit forms of health-care delivery predominated under the auspices of charitable and religious institutions. Medical staffs influenced hospital policy and had free reign in the clinical realm.[5]

By increasing access to medical care through broad-based insurance coverage, federal programs improved opportunities for commercial investment in health-care delivery systems. Once commercial investors gained a foothold, they sought economies of scale. Corporate purchasers of hospitals consolidated their holdings, integrating hospitals and related facilities. After their initial appearance in 1968, investor-owned hospital chains expanded rapidly. By 1985 just four companies owned or managed 12 percent of all

U.S. hospitals.[6] Responding to pressures to cut costs, hospital mergers multiplied during the 1990s.[7]

Physicians shared in these profit-making ventures. Although physician ownership of hospitals declined following government involvement in health care, physician investment increased in diagnostic imaging centers, clinical laboratories, medical equipment suppliers, freestanding surgical centers, nursing homes, and other ancillary facilities. By the early 1990s physicians owned shares in 25 to 80 percent of ancillary medical facilities, depending on the region and type of facility. Corporate consolidation of the health-care industry made this possible. Large hospital chains formed joint ventures with physician groups or established limited partnerships that included physician investors. Because most patients had insurance coverage, and state laws sheltered investors from liability, the risks of ownership were minimal.[8]

As long as the nation experienced strong economic growth and relatively low rates of inflation, social programs like Medicare continued to expand. These favorable economic conditions disappeared after the 1960s. In the 1970s economic growth slowed but inflation rates soared, particularly in health care. In the 1980s continued funding of social programs became more problematic when federal and many state governments experienced large budget deficits.[9] The usual response to these economic events was retrenchment of social programs through cost containment. Government officials attempted to control costs by enhancing market competition, monitoring expenditures, and pursuing fraudulent practices. These efforts signaled the end of the medical profession's monopoly over the medical field.

Breaking Up the Medical Monopoly

Schattschneider observed that "the attempt to control the scope of conflict has a bearing on federal-state-local relations, for one way to restrict the scope of conflict is to *localize* it, while one way to expand it is to nationalize it."[10] Until the 1970s the medical profession had been successful in channeling conflict through local institutions, such as county medical societies and community hospitals. These institutions invoked norms and ethics that maintained traditional bonds between physicians and their patients, discouraged competition, and supported fee-for-service medicine. Courts preserved local self-governance through the corporate practice of medicine doctrine, the locality rule in medical malpractice cases, and the "learned professions" exemption in antitrust actions.

If market competition was to succeed as a means of controlling costs, federal officials had to overcome these institutional and legal barriers. Heeding Schattschneider's advice, the Federal Trade Commission and other agencies of the federal government sought to nationalize the scope of conflict. Application of the antitrust laws to the medical field through the federal courts was a principal means of doing this. In the process, federal policy undermined traditional means of regulating physician behavior. When local institutions faltered, state and federal agencies took up the slack.

With few exceptions, federal antitrust actions against the medical profession did not succeed until the 1970s.[11] Courts originally took the position that federal laws did not apply because the practice of medicine was local in character. Professional activities, courts once said, neither affected interstate commerce nor did they constitute a "trade" for purposes of the Sherman Antitrust Act.[12] Many judges also believed, for policy reasons, that "noncommercial" professional activities should be exempt from federal antitrust scrutiny.[13]

According to Jeffrey Berlant, "the most plausible source for an explanation of the rise of the medical profession and of the professions in general in the United States lies in the political conflict between local and national economic interests."[14] Local economic interests deployed several weapons in their war against national corporations. Among these were state laws, including those on occupational licensure, that deterred outsiders from disrupting local economies. Another was the Sherman Antitrust Act which targeted national monopolies while leaving local monopolies intact. Legal doctrines, such as that exempting "learned professions" from antitrust scrutiny, favored local interests, as did narrow interpretations of the Commerce Clause and of the "trade" or "commerce" provisions in the Sherman Act.

When the federal government turned the spotlight on local monopolies in the 1970s, the medical profession was among those that received intense scrutiny. Much of the initial focus was on medical licensure laws. Government studies, as well as some by noted lawyers and economists, showed that such laws created shortages among health-care personnel, inhibited geographic and career mobility, and prevented the development of more cost-effective means of providing medical care.[15] These studies persuaded federal officials that greater uniformity in medical licensure and discipline was necessary. Federal officials called for national standards but ultimately chose to work with state authorities rather than impose a national licensure scheme.[16]

In 1975 the Federal Trade Commission (FTC) created a task force to consider the preemption of state laws governing occupational licensure.[17]

Potentially blocking implementation of FTC plans was the Supreme Court's decision in *Parker v. Brown* (1942),[18] holding that state activities were immune from federal antitrust scrutiny. The implications of the "state action" doctrine for the FTC's preemptive authority under its enabling statute was unclear. In 1977 the Court provided further guidance in *Bates v. State Bar of Arizona* (1977),[19] when it applied the state action doctrine to disciplinary rules prohibiting lawyer advertising. Although the Court struck down the rules on First Amendment grounds, it reaffirmed *Parker* by precluding any claim against Arizona under the Sherman Act.

Deterred from acting against state medical boards directly, the FTC pursued the AMA. In a 1979 order, the FTC prohibited restrictions on advertising, solicitation, and various contractual and fee arrangements.[20] The FTC was on solid ground, following the Supreme Court's ruling in *Goldfarb v. Virginia State Bar* (1975),[21] rejecting the antitrust exemption for "noncommercial" professional practices. After numerous appeals, the FTC's 1979 order remained intact.[22] Under its terms, the AMA had to amend its Principles of Medical Ethics and sever all ties for one year with any state or local medical society that engaged in prohibited activities.

Disciplinary activities of state and local medical societies, including the resolution of patient grievances, "virtually stopped in most areas" after the Supreme Court affirmed the FTC order. Fear of litigation was the reason for the low level of activity. The AMA reported that from 1982 to 1987, either the FTC, the Department of Justice, or another government agency investigated ten state societies and thirteen county societies. During that period, disgruntled member or nonmember physicians sued ten state societies and twenty county societies for alleged antitrust violations.[23]

Federal officials required the AMA and various state societies to strike "anticompetitive" provisions from professional codes. State and local medical societies suspended efforts to regulate overcharging, fee splitting, contract practice, advertising, and other forms of "unfair" competition. Taking action proved risky without direct state supervision. For all practical purposes, professional organizations lost the authority to effectively regulate their own membership or to mediate disputes among physicians and their patients. In Baltimore, where the local medical society had been active in resolving patient grievances, the situation was much the same. As reflected in table 1.1, the Baltimore City Medical Society resolved over 150 cases a year by 1973. In the late 1970s these efforts ceased. Despite the fact that medical societies could still muster solid legal grounds for mediating patient complaints, the risks and costs of litigation were too great.

Although the inability to adjust patient grievances was troubling, the medical profession was also concerned about the effect of antitrust laws on physician peer review. Peer review was the principal mechanism for determining staff privileges in hospitals and for monitoring and evaluating physician performance. The American College of Surgeons commenced peer review in 1918 to assess the quality of candidates for board certification. In 1952 the Joint Commission on Accreditation of Hospitals incorporated peer review in its standards for hospitals seeking accreditation. Reliance on peer review for monitoring physician performance steadily increased with changes in the medical field.[24]

Following passage of Medicare and resulting cost-containment initiatives, pressures on peer reviewers mounted. For physicians, an adverse peer review decision meant losing not only hospital privileges but also eligibility under government and private insurance programs. Trends favoring more physicians and fewer hospitals increased competition for hospital affiliation, raising the stakes even higher.[25] Yet, legal challenges to decisions of medical staff were infrequent until the mid-1970s. This changed when the Supreme Court rejected the "learned professions" exemption in *Goldfarb* and relaxed the connection between interstate commerce and the local practice of medicine.[26]

Physicians denied staff privileges could now sue in federal court, alleging violations of federal antitrust law. Lawsuits by physicians against physicians, the AMA reported in 1988, "account for the largest percentage of antitrust cases involving the health care field."[27] Courts applied a "rule-of-reason" approach to privilege denials that required balancing the procompetitive and anticompetitive effects of medical staff decisions. Lacking clear legal standards, hospital boards were hesitant to implement adverse credentialing decisions.[28]

Despite limited chances of success at trial, physicians who challenged privilege denials held a strategic advantage. Simply threatening suit was often sufficient to provoke a favorable settlement because of the enormous costs involved in defending antitrust cases and the potential for large jury awards. Physicians denied privileges could sue for treble damages and attorneys' fees. Hospitals sought to reduce the threat of antitrust litigation through oversight of decision making by medical staff. Attorneys and administrators assumed prominent roles in decisions that were once the sole province of doctors. As one commentator predicted in 1982, antitrust litigation "could turn the hospital into a public utility that grants admitting privileges to all health practitioners who are competent within the terms of their licenses."[29]

The Supreme Court rocked the medical community in 1988 when it reinstated $2.2 million in antitrust treble damages awarded in the case of *Patrick v. Burget.*[30] As often occurs in celebrated cases, the facts were somewhat unique. Substantial evidence supported Patrick's contention that competing physicians had acted in bad faith in revoking his privileges at the only hospital in a small Oregon community. But the Ninth Circuit Court of Appeals reversed a jury verdict in favor of Patrick on grounds that the state action doctrine protected peer review at Oregon hospitals.

The Supreme Court disagreed with the Ninth Circuit's application of the state action doctrine to the facts of the case. For state action immunity to apply, the Court emphasized, there had to be a clearly articulated state policy supporting the challenged activities coupled with active state supervision. In *Patrick,* the Court found that the second prong of the test, active state supervision, was lacking. It was not enough, the Court said, that state agencies monitor actions of peer review bodies through reporting procedures. Active state supervision required state officials to directly oversee the peer review process and correct abuses if necessary.

By making self-regulation a hazardous activity, antitrust actions altered the relationship between private and public authorities. If medical societies were to continue their involvement in physician discipline, they now required protection under the "state action" doctrine. Private medical societies that wanted to remain active in physician discipline had to become agents of the state. Federally sponsored peer review organizations and state medical boards, not state and local medical societies, would be responsible for investigating complaints for incompetence and unprofessional conduct. As indicated in figure 2.1, board actions increased following the decline of grievance committees of local and state medical societies in the 1970s. Even more telling, board actions against physicians for incompetence increased sharply following antitrust actions against credentialing committees of hospital boards in the 1980s.

Linking Medical Malpractice and Physician Discipline

In the absence of government regulation, the public's principal means of recourse against poorly performing physicians were lawsuits for malpractice. Lawsuits were relatively rare before the 1960s, as were disciplinary actions. Both increased for many of the same reasons—improved access to health care, a more complex technology, rising consumer expectations, and the decline of the professional order.[31] Just as federal courts struck down legal barriers to antitrust actions against local medical societies and community hospitals, so state courts removed legal impediments to professional liability. Court doctrines, such as "informed consent," "common knowledge," and "res ipsa loquitur," made it easier for plaintiffs to prove their cases. Many courts also curtailed application of the locality rule, furthering a trend toward uniformity in medical practice.[32]

Enhanced litigation and large jury awards led to so-called crises in the availability and affordability of malpractice insurance during the 1970s and 1980s. Several insurance companies stopped covering physicians for malpractice, while others sharply increased their premiums. Reacting to these events, organized medicine pressed state legislatures to curb litigation by passing laws that made it harder for plaintiffs to sue and to recover damages against physicians. Among the reforms physicians sought were restrictions on attorneys fees, limits on the amount of damages that juries could award for pain and suffering, and the reversal of court doctrines that lowered the burden of proof.[33]

Although many states agreed to reform their laws on professional liability, they exacted a price from organized medicine for their cooperation. That price was closer scrutiny of physicians for malpractice and other asserted misdeeds.[34] Several states, including California, Oregon, and Massachusetts, enacted legislation in the 1970s that reorganized board operations and expanded board powers. California added eight members to its board in 1975, six of them from the general public. Legislators in California also split the board into three semi-autonomous divisions, each having separate responsibility for licensing, discipline, and allied health professionals.[35] Oregon, along with California and several other states, required insurance carriers and physicians to report malpractice cases to the state medical board. To encourage reporting, Oregon assured confidentiality and provided immunity from civil lawsuits.[36] In 1975 Massachusetts appointed an entirely new board and established three-member tribunals, each consisting of a trial judge, a physician, and an attorney, to hear cases of physician malpractice.[37]

Most states attacked the problem of physician discipline in different ways, but four areas received widespread attention. First, the composition of board panels changed to reflect consumer interests. Second, state medical societies lost some of their authority over the selection of physician members to board panels. Third, boards assumed responsibility for investigating a wide range of complaints, including those for medical malpractice. Fourth, states gained oversight of board operations through sunset laws and centralization of administrative functions. Taken together, these trends indicated a diminished role for organized medicine and an enhanced role for state governments in medical discipline.

Changing the composition of board panels was a significant step toward severing ties with organized medicine. The U.S. Supreme Court rejected equal protection and due process challenges to board composition in *Gibson v. Berryhill* (1973)[38] and *Friedman v. Rodgers* (1979).[39] Both cases involved turf battles between rival optometric associations. Despite allegations of bias and conflict of interest, the Court refused to enter the fray, as did state courts faced with similar complaints.[40] Because courts signaled that they would give professions great leeway in resolving issues related to state licensing boards, consumer groups and others seeking to enhance discipline looked to state legislatures and governors' offices for relief.

The percentage of physicians on board panels slowly, but steadily, declined after California became the first state to appoint a layperson to its medical board in 1961. Figure 2.2 reflects changes in the composition of board panels for available years. In 1941, the year that Nebraska's state medical association canvassed state medical practice acts, physicians comprised 94 percent of all board members. By 1976, the year that Frank Grad and Noelia Marti began their study of state medical boards for the federal government, physician members had declined to 83 percent, while public members had climbed to 10 percent.[41] When the Federation of State Medical Boards began compiling detailed information on board operations around 1987, physician members comprised 78 percent of board panels, and public members comprised over 17 percent.[42] In 1996 physicians represented 74 percent of all board members, while public members accounted for almost 21 percent.

As demonstrated in figure 2.2, most boards had at least one or two public members by 1987. Despite their initial opposition, many physicians believed that public members would enhance the profession's poor image. Addressing the federation's annual business meeting in 1975, Howard Horns of Minnesota claimed that "public members might provide a communication channel and prevent a great deal of misunderstanding and suspicion."[43] Those seeking structural reforms questioned whether such "token" representation would make any difference.[44] Although researchers Grad and Marti argued that lay membership would "insure impartiality and greater public accountability,"[45] early indications suggested that such optimism was unfounded. Based on case studies from 1960 to 1977, Andrew Dolan and Nicole Urban found that board "effectiveness," measured in terms of the number of disciplinary actions taken, failed "to respond to changes in nonphysician dominance of boards."[46] It would take more than a few public members for boards to increase the number of disciplinary actions.

Another change concerned the attenuated role of state medical societies in selecting physicians to serve on board panels. Medical societies his-

FIGURE 2.2

Member composition of state medical board panels, 1941–1996.

Source: Data from Nebraska Survey (1941); Grad and Marti, *Physicians' Licensure and Discipline*, 370–83; Federation of State Medical Boards, *Exchange* (1987): 45, (1995–96): 4–5.

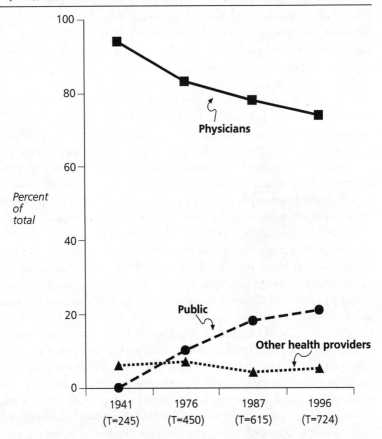

torically played a large role in the selection process; in some states, such as Alabama, Maryland, and North Carolina, legislatures delegated the power of appointment to the state medical society.[47] A more common method was for governors to appoint members from society-approved lists. Writing in the late 1960s, Derbyshire lamented that "medical societies can exercise so much influence in the appointment of quasi-judicial boards which are arms of the state governments." Derbyshire noted that state societies often nominated candidates for political reasons rather than choosing the best person for the job. Medical societies, he said, "frequently ignored professional and educational attributes, endorsing some faithful political stalwart who has worked his way up in the councils of his society."[48] Derbyshire's findings tracked those contained in the 1961 report of the AMA's Medical Disciplinary Committee.[49]

Starting in the 1960s, several states changed their laws to reduce the role of medical societies in nominating candidates for appointment to state medical boards. In 1976 medical societies in thirty states nominated candidates for gubernatorial appointment.[50] By 1986 medical societies in only nineteen states retained an exclusive role in the nomination process. According to information compiled by the Federation of State Medical Boards, little changed between 1986 and 1996.[51] These findings do not reflect the indirect influence that state societies had on executive appointments. Nevertheless, the overall picture indicates that organized medicine lost ground to competing interests.

The malpractice crises also forced boards to take on new responsibilities. Many states passed laws that required hospitals, insurance companies, professional associations, and other entities to report malpractice and other violations involving physicians to state boards. Table 2.2 shows the total number of states that required entities to report violations for the years 1976, 1986, and 1996. Although laws differed among states, the trend favored mandatory reporting, particularly for hospitals, liability insurance carriers, medical societies, and licensed physicians.

Laws that required individuals and entities to report physician misconduct were not self-executing. Physicians were reluctant to report their colleagues, and hospitals often allowed physicians to resign voluntarily to avoid reporting them to state boards.[52] To encourage reporting, medical practice acts assured confidentiality and provided immunity from prosecution to individuals who reported violations in good faith. In some instances, states authorized boards to fine those who failed to report.[53]

Reporting requirements significantly increased the number of complaints that boards had to screen and resolve. Oregon's board experienced a "three-to-four-fold increase" in the volume of complaints against practitioners in the ten years following the enactment of its mandatory reporting laws in 1977 and 1978.[54] The caseload of Maryland's board increased from 735 to 1,245 between 1986 and 1987, after the passage of similar legislation.[55] This massive transfer of complaints from the private sector to state boards and from other government agencies to state boards caused huge backlogs and delays. State medical boards were under enormous pressure to respond, but they had neither the resources nor the organization to manage their growing caseloads.

TABLE 2.2

Individuals and Other Entities Required to Report Possible
Violations to State Medical Boards, 1976, 1986, and 1996

	1976	1986	1996
All licensees	6	25	36
Licensee committing a violation	1	16	28
Courts	10	16	20
Hospitals (staff and administrators)	16	39	50
Liability insurance carrier(s)	20	27	42
Local medical osteopathic societies	14	22	33
Local professional societies	*	14	30
Other state agencies	1	10	15
State / local law enforcement agencies	0	6	12
State medical / osteopathic societies	14	22	35
State professional / speciality societies	*	15	32
Professional / peer review organizations	0	1	21
Physicians treating physicians for special disorders	5	1	12
Other health-care professions	1	2	11
Federal agencies	0	1	2

Source: Data from Grad and Marti, *Physicians' Licensure and Discipline*, 384–91; the Federation of State Medical Boards, *Exchange* (1986): 24, (1995–96): 38–39.

Note: For comparative purposes, only allopathic medical boards for each of the fifty states and the District of Columbia are included.

*Information not available.

In particular, boards did not know what to do with the large number of malpractice cases that arrived at their doorstep. Many boards, like New Jersey's, almost ignored them.[56] Leading physicians, such as AMA President James Todd, believed that boards should not equate lawsuits for malpractice, often brought against capable physicians, with physician incompetence. According to Todd, "isolated incidents of malpractice action bear little, if any, relationship to competence or impairment."[57] James Kusserow, Inspector General for the U.S. Department of Health and Human Services, apparently agreed. In an appearance before the annual meeting of the Federation of State Medical Boards in 1987, Kusserow remarked, "I don't know what our office could ever do with that information. I'm not sure of its relevance and don't know how it could be used as a predictor of future conduct or behavior."[58]

The frequent inability of boards to address their newfound responsibilities caused states to search for ways to enhance board performance. Between 1976 and 1981, thirty-five states passed sunset laws to assess board activity on a regular basis.[59] Boards continued to function but came under intense scrutiny from politicians and the media.[60] Although some called for the elimination of physician membership on board panels and secrecy in board investigations, no state went that far.[61] Rather, many states weakened relations between boards and organized medicine by consolidating board operations through an executive department of state government.

States had several options for making boards more efficient. They could assume certain housekeeping and administrative functions, such as the purchase of supplies or the collection of licensing fees. They could go a step further and seize control of budgetary, staffing, and investigative functions. They could even require boards to submit all policy decisions, including proposed disciplinary actions, to a central agency for review and implementation. As a final step, states could simply delegate the authority for making final decisions in disciplinary matters to another agency of state government, as New York did in 1975.[62]

Although few states followed New York's lead, several states tightened their control of board operations during the 1970s and 1980s through government reorganization. Most states simply provided administrative, fiscal, and budgetary assistance, but the potential for further action always existed.[63] For boards to remain independent, they had to command the resources required to manage a growing caseload. Building a modern state medical board to manage political conflict as well as medical discipline was the paramount challenge.

Consumerism and the New Regulatory Framework

Public discontent with the medical profession did not disappear after organized medicine formed grievance committees in the 1950s. It continued to grow in the 1960s and 1970s.[64] By the 1980s consumer organizations such as SHAME (Stop Hospital and Medical Errors), Public Citizen, and the Citizen Advocacy Center were quite active. The federal government, through the Office of the Inspector General for the Department of Health and Human Services, frequently scrutinized board activities and reported to Congress on board performance.[65] Hearings before Congress in 1984, 1986, and 1990 placed physician discipline on the national agenda.[66] Just as Schattschneider had predicted, organized medicine was no longer able to contain the conflict once the "wider public" became involved.

Before changes in medical and information technology revolutionized medical practice, physicians usually treated patients in their own offices, combining their best medical judgment with an intimate understanding of their patients' backgrounds. Years of medical training gave physicians the knowledge patients lacked to make appropriate decisions about their own medical care. Because of the inequality of knowledge, the physician-patient relationship was built on trust. To safeguard patients from abuse, the medical profession required that physicians heed a strict moral or ethical code.[67]

By the 1980s forces sustaining the traditional physician-patient relationship and the accompanying ethical code were in disarray. Structural change weakened private institutions that were responsible for establishing norms, enforcing codes of professional conduct, and maintaining competence. State and local medical societies remained the backbone of organized medicine, but incentives to join these organizations decreased after government and corporations entered the medical field. Benefits of society membership at one time included malpractice coverage, patient referrals and consultations, hospital access, and professional appointments. Most of these benefits were now available to physicians without having to join their state or local medical societies. Managed-care organizations, for example, often provided professional liability insurance and long-term disability coverage.[68] These organizations also determined the nature and extent of professional contacts and patient referrals for participating physicians.[69]

The profession's ability to gauge physician competence also suffered. Medical schools doubled class sizes, and large numbers of foreign-trained physicians joined the workforce in the 1970s and 1980s.[70] During congressional hearings on the Health Care Quality Improvement Act of 1986, experts testified that 118,000 physicians, or about one-fifth of physicians practicing in the United States, had never attended a medical school accredited by the Liaison Committee on Medical Education.[71] Medical staff of hospitals lacked the leverage to regulate incompetent practitioners. Antitrust actions had weakened their resolve, and hospital administrators had co-opted their authority. Hospitals themselves became victims of structural change. Because managed care emphasized the prevention of disease over its cure as a means of cutting costs, it shifted the setting for patient services. Insurers preferred less expensive ambulatory care centers and home-health agencies to hospitals for surgical treatment and follow-up care. When hospitalization was necessary, HMOs pressured physicians to reduce the number of days patients could stay in hospitals following treatment. Occupancy rates declined, and many hospitals closed.[72]

After more than a century of decentralized control under the auspices of solo practitioners, the medical field achieved corporate integration.[73] The market became the preferred mechanism for allocating medical services, reducing costs, and determining quality. Physicians were "providers" of medical care, as were hospitals and other health-care professionals; patients were "consumers." The role of government was to monitor the performance of providers and to furnish sufficient information so that consumers could make informed choices about which providers afforded competent care.[74] State medical boards were a potential source of information, as were federally sponsored peer review organizations and law enforcement agencies of federal and state governments.

During the 1980s consumers increasingly looked to state medical boards to take appropriate action against poorly performing physicians. Rising levels of education, greater availability of information through the use of computers, increasing complexity of medical practice, and a growing number of paraprofessional workers reduced the so-called knowledge gap between physicians and consumers.[75] Individual physicians no longer sustained a monopoly over a specific body of knowledge. Consumers reasonably demanded a partnership role in their care and treatment. Likewise, they expected government agencies, such as state medical boards, to protect them from physicians who abused drugs, had sex with their patients, and were incompetent.

According to historian Samuel Hays, consumer interests disrupted an older regulatory framework that was limited to resolving conflicts among producers. The new form of regulation combined market enterprise with regulatory agencies that countenanced consumer values.[76] Mark Yessian, Regional Inspector General for the Department of Health and Human Services, proclaimed the demise of self-regulation due to consumer pressures for more public accountability. He called on boards to abandon their ties to the medical profession and to protect the public. Yessian admonished board members who were physicians to set aside their professional interests in favor of their official responsibilities. A change in the "mind-set" of physicians concerning medical regulation, Yessian argued, was required to accommodate a "patient-driven" health-care system.[77] With the decline of the professional order, the responsibility for protecting consumers fell squarely on government entities such as state medical boards. Their roles more clearly defined, boards emerged as the primary public authorities for disciplining wayward physicians.

Conclusion

During the 1970s and 1980s, medical discipline gained a prominent place on the national agenda. The reasons for this were complex and often had little to do with the poor performance of physicians. Rather, the rising costs of health care and problems related to crises in the availability and affordability of insurance for medical malpractice heightened concerns over professional accountability. Efforts to resolve these dilemmas undermined traditional means of regulating physician behavior. Using market competition to control costs, the federal government opened the door to antitrust actions against local medical societies and peer review bodies of private hospitals. Reacting to medical malpractice crises in the 1970s and the 1980s, state governments took action to dissolve long-standing ties between boards and organized medicine.

Once in the public realm, medical discipline achieved new standing. As Schattschneider recognized, "inevitably the outcome of a contest is controlled by the level at which the decision is made."[78] Placing decision-making authority in the hands of state medical boards widened the scope of conflict. Federal and state agencies, politicians, the media, and consumer groups pressed boards to prosecute cases they had neither the resources nor the tools to handle. Some cases involved unethical conduct that professional societies formerly resolved through mediation. Other cases dealt with medical malpractice that courts and arbitration panels pursued through a complex legal process that utilized formal rules and procedures.

Despite their inadequacies, boards had little choice but to move forward. Laws that required health-care providers and entities to report physician misconduct made boards the cornerstone of the disciplinary process. States signaled their readiness to take control if physicians failed to respond. Faced with public demands that they improve their performance, boards evolved into complex organizations that kept physicians in power but relied on bureaucratic management to expedite the handling of complaints.

CHAPTER THREE

Building a Modern State Medical Board

Overcoming entrenched interests and past practices was a distinct challenge. Boards entered the modern era hampered by limited funds, staff, and information. If boards were to protect the public through the efficient and orderly prosecution of physicians for incompetence and unprofessional conduct, they required the support of both government and organized medicine. Boards faced the problem of gaining the assistance of state agencies and organized medicine without sacrificing operational autonomy.

Central to the struggle between public and professional interests was the means that boards used to resolve complaints about physician performance. Before the 1970s most boards resolved complaints using a professional model of decision making. The attributes of the professional model included collegiality, informality, and confidentiality.[1] These attributes reflected physicians' attitudes toward their work, specifically their insistence on independent judgment and freedom from outside control. Only physicians were competent to judge other physicians, and only physicians acting collectively could take disciplinary action. Physicians eschewed formal rules, hierarchy, and external assistance. They pursued neither funding nor personnel to advance government regulation of the medical profession. Rather, physicians entrusted private organizations, such as local medical societies and community hospitals, with the enforcement of professional norms and standards.

State governments offered an alternative framework that stressed hierarchy, formality, and accountability. By making the process for disciplining physicians more bureaucratic, government officials hoped to oversee board operations and to improve board performance. Keys to rationalizing case management were the introduction of information systems, the coordination of resources and personnel, and the use of trained staff and standardized procedures for categorizing, investigating, and resolving complaints. Reconciling the two approaches challenged all concerned. Although crucial for coordinating and supervising large organizations, hierarchy jeopardized collegial relations and threatened professional autonomy. Formal rules and procedures promoted uniformity and predictability but limited flexibility and professional discretion. Public access to records and proceedings furthered consumer knowledge but inhibited candid peer review.

Boards struggled to resolve the contradictions between these two models during the 1970s and 1980s. The extent to which boards succeeded or failed often depended on state and local politics and, in particular, on media coverage and the role of organized medicine. Some states, such as California, New York, and New Jersey, reorganized their boards in the 1970s in response to the crisis in medical malpractice insurance. Other states, such as Maryland and Massachusetts, waited until the 1980s before making significant changes. Still others continued the slow, but steady, process of incremental reform.[2] Ultimately the real issue was who would control medical discipline—would it be state governments, organized medicine, or boards themselves?

The Professional Model and the Disciplinary Process

Many observers and analysts blamed inadequate staffing and insufficient funds for the lack of disciplinary actions against licensed physicians.[3] They assumed that the failure of state governments to supply these ingredients prevented boards from moving forward. Although it was certainly true that limited resources constrained board productivity, state and local medical societies were not particularly interested in furthering board powers to discipline physicians before the 1980s.[4] So long as professional societies and medical staff of hospitals exerted control, medical discipline was self-contained. Formal discipline at the state level came at the expense of the medical profession because it expanded conflict into the public realm. Seeking to contain the scope of conflict, physicians stressed informality, collegiality, and confidentiality in the decision-making process. These were the founding principles of board structure and operation.

Three trends threatened to undermine these founding principles. First, changes in legal process made disciplinary proceedings more formal, requiring boards to seek legal assistance and to revise their procedures for resolving complaints. Second, the number of complaints that boards received significantly increased in the 1970s and 1980s, straining the capacity of physicians, who served on boards as volunteers, to manage an expanding workload. Third, the need for boards to report their findings, coupled with the passage of laws expanding public access to records and meetings, heightened exposure to media and consumer organizations.

When dealing with their fellow colleagues, most physicians preferred to proceed informally. "Doctors," Phillip Wylie observed, "are busy people. They hate committees. They hate litigation. They hate to interfere with each other, lest they be interfered with."[5] Hospitals, medical societies, and medical boards resolved most matters without taking formal action.[6] State medical boards, for instance, often met informally with licensees to discuss possible misconduct.[7] This usually ended the matter or resulted in an informal letter of reprimand, a letter of admonishment, or a letter to cease and desist from offensive activities. Boards typically resolved about five to ten cases informally for every formal sanction.[8]

Legal process changed the way that boards functioned by curtailing the direct involvement of board members in case dispositions. During the 1960s administrative agencies adopted procedural rules and regulations in response to civil rights and civil liberties violations by government officials. Curtailing official discretion through legal process, they argued, was the best way to prevent abuse. Advocates of legal process claimed that closer adherence to procedural and evidentiary rules guaranteed more fairness in agency decision making. Courts themselves were in the vanguard of the movement, reversing agency decisions that failed to afford due process. According to attorney Philip K. Howard, "the simple 'notice and comment' requirement of the Administrative Procedure Act had become, by judicial fiat, a celebration of extensive process."[9]

Few board members were eager to devote attention to procedural details, but courts were not about to ignore such matters. Before the Supreme Court's holding in *Schware v. Board of Bar Examiners* in 1957,[10] there had been general agreement that a license to practice a chosen occupation was a privilege, not a right protected by the Fourteenth Amendment. In *Schware* the Court rejected the right-privilege distinction in cases involving occupational licensure, holding that due process protections applied to the granting and revocation of licenses. The door was now open for courts to determine how much process was actually due.

Several components of the disciplinary process occupied the attention of state appellate courts during the 1960s and 1970s. These included the procedural and evidentiary rules governing board hearings, the specificity of charges, the right to counsel, and the impartiality of decision makers.[11] Speaking before delegates to the annual meeting of the Federation of State Medical Boards in 1962, Delaware Judge Charles L. Terry Jr. favored "all of the major safeguards," including "full notice, right to counsel, right to production of all evidence, right to subpoena, right to examination of all witnesses, right to be judged by competent judges from among ones 'peers,' right to appeal, right to review."[12] Although state administrative procedure acts and court rulings did not force boards to adhere to strict judicial requirements, the procedures that boards now had to follow were considerably more burdensome than they had been only a few years earlier.[13] Complicating the matter further were the harshness of available sanctions,[14] the ambiguity or inconsistency of grounds for disciplining physicians, judicial reversal or stay of board actions,[15] and difficulties in meeting the burden of proof.[16] Under the circumstances, a physician's conduct had to be particularly egregious to evoke formal charges.

Until boards learned to play the game under a new set of rules, the number of cases they resolved would not increase. For physicians serving as board members, requirements of due process constrained prehearing activity. Being triers of fact, board members could neither contact offenders before initiating formal charges nor have so-called *ex parte* conversations with them after bringing formal charges. To resolve most cases, board members had to rely on intermediaries for investigation, settlement, and prosecution.[17] They needed adequate staff to review complaints, obtain and evaluate medical records, and interview witnesses. They also needed attorneys to advise them on legal matters and to negotiate settlements. Bureaucratic and legal entanglements made it difficult for physicians active in private practice to retain their former hands-on style.

Another threat to the professional model stemmed from backlogged cases. Collegial decision making was a time-consuming and cumbersome process. For several reasons, board meetings were not a good forum for adversarial hearings. The orderly and efficient introduction of evidence required a unitary decision maker familiar with legal technicalities. Although many boards had the assistance of legal counsel, physicians who chaired hearings made important evidentiary rulings. Board members did not sit as a jury, so few could resist the temptation to become part of the proceedings, delaying the outcome. Consistency was another problem. Boards seldom convened more than once or twice a month, making it difficult to address complex cases involving multiple witnesses and documents. When boards met, their agenda encompassed numerous items, some quite pressing. Hearings were often the last items on board agendas and, if not completed, were resumed at later meetings. Lengthy interruptions in the presentation of evidence created problems for all concerned—board members, attorneys, and witnesses. Board members had to reacquaint themselves with the evidence, and attorneys and witnesses had to prepare and to adjust their schedules accordingly.[18]

Boards had to either limit the type and amount of complaints they would consider or develop alternative techniques for resolving cases. The former was not a viable option. Boards' jurisdiction was expanding, not contracting, because of the consumer movement, mandated reporting of malpractice cases, and federal antitrust actions against state and local medical societies. As part-time volunteers, board members were incapable of managing a growing caseload on their own. To expedite hearings, board members had to delegate decision-making authority to others. By the mid-1970s relief was in sight: laws in twenty-five states allowed hearing officers to conduct evidentiary hearings on behalf of medical boards.[19] By 1986 laws in thirty- six states permitted the use of hearing officers.[20] Board members still had the final word on most disciplinary matters, but attorneys, hearing officers, and case managers now came between them and the physicians they regulated.

The final threat to the professional model came from media and consumer organizations seeking to publicize physician misconduct. As the AMA discovered in the 1950s, information concerning disciplinary activities of state medical boards was in short supply, and what existed was difficult to obtain. The AMA's problems were minor compared to those of media and consumer groups that were on the outside looking in. Board parochialism and poor record keeping were principal reasons for the AMA's woes, but media and consumer groups faced additional obstacles, including laws protecting the confidentiality of medical records and board deliberations. Public Citizen reportedly encountered organized resistance from Maryland's medical society in seeking to publish the first consumer's directory of local physicians in 1974. According to the directory's authors: "Most people can find out more about a car they plan to buy than they can about a doctor who may hold their life in his or her hands."[21]

Enactment by most states of freedom of information acts and open meetings laws in the 1960s and 1970s signaled a trend toward a more open system of government. Media and consumer interests employed these new tools in seeking access to disciplinary records and board deliberations.[22] By and large, they were unsuccessful. Courts limited the inspection of board records to those parties actually involved in specific cases.[23] State laws carved out similar exceptions.[24] Unless boards issued final orders detailing their findings, the public had little knowledge of poorly performing physicians. The reasons for continued secrecy varied. According to one commentator, "The scales have been weighted toward secrecy on the unstated assumption that professionals have higher morals and deserve by virtue of their standing in society to be given the benefit of the doubt."[25] The Office of Inspector General for the Department of Health and Human Services suggested that boards often avoided formal hearings by entering into consent agreements with physicians that kept disciplinary actions confidential.[26]

Despite these setbacks, the "closed society" that physicians had formed and maintained since the early twentieth century was crumbling.[27] The real breach came in 1986 when Congress passed legislation establishing a national practitioners data bank to collect reports of disciplinary actions taken by hospitals, professional societies, malpractice insurers, and state medical boards.[28] Congress intended that the data bank aid licensing and credentialing authorities in detecting and monitoring the interstate movements of problem physicians.[29] Because boards were inconsistent in reporting disciplinary actions to a central clearinghouse, physicians disciplined in one state continued practicing by simply moving to another.

Although Congress excluded consumers from among the list of groups and individuals given access to information on medical discipline, the mere existence of a federal data bank accelerated efforts by boards and organized medicine to develop alternative systems. For example, the Federation of State Medical Boards unveiled its Disciplinary Data Bank around 1985, as federal legislation was under consideration. During congressional hearings, the federation sought to postpone implementation of the federal data bank, claiming that a national program was premature.[30] The AMA adopted a similar stance, arguing that a federal repository would be "susceptible to abuses and breaches of confidentiality."[31] In 1986 the AMA's House of Delegates moved to expand its Physician Masterfile to provide additional guidance on the credentialing of physicians.[32] According to AMA President John Tupper, "The fact is that in this era of increased accountability something *like* the data bank is *going* to be out there. So we've got to make sure that the profession identifies *who* and *what* the bad apples in medicine *are,* or they will *spoil* the glorious reputation this profession has built for itself."[33]

Despite limitations on public access to disciplinary records, the movement for more disclosure was now irreversible. Pressures on boards to report their findings substantially increased the amount of material available to media and consumer groups. By the early 1990s Public Citizen had collected sufficient information to begin publishing individual state listings of problem physicians.[34] It was only a matter of time before advances in technology made information on physicians' backgrounds even more accessible to consumers.[35]

Government Efforts to Reorganize Board Operations

Boards could not continue to decide cases utilizing the professional model of decision making. It lacked formality, delayed the resolution of complaints, and hindered efforts to publicize disciplinary actions. Government agencies offered a more bureaucratic framework that incorporated legal process, standardized case review, and stressed public accountability, all of which were foreign to physicians who lived in a world in which informal relationships and independent judgment prevailed.[36] As sociologist

Eliot Freidson pointed out, the "'macro' or policy-oriented perspective [of administrators was] quite different from the 'micro' or clinical practice perspective of rank and file practitioners trying to cope with everyday problems of work."[37] Improving board performance was not simply a matter of gaining additional resources. Before medical discipline could proceed on a larger scale, changes had to take place in how physicians related to one another and to governmental authority.

As we have seen, state efforts to reorganize board operations occurred in response to crises in the availability and affordability of medical malpractice insurance. During the 1970s most states altered board size and composition; many states consolidated board operations. The Office of Inspector General for the Department of Health and Human Services reported that the number of boards under the control of an umbrella agency increased from sixteen in 1969 to thirty-one in 1986.[38] These efforts widened the scope of conflict as many boards, for the first time, experienced diffuse pressures to discipline physicians for a variety of offenses.

Despite these changes, overall board performance failed to improve because physicians had not yet reconciled professional and bureaucratic models of decision making. Stated another way, the conflicting tendencies toward the privatization and the socialization of conflict destabilized medical discipline during the 1970s and early 1980s. Physicians did not want additional resources for disciplining fellow colleagues unless they could control them. As early as 1956, the Federation of State Medical Boards made its position clear concerning state takeover of board operations:

> There is a trend to streamline government with the result that licensing boards and agencies are abolished with responsibilities placed in large, multipurpose political departments of government with all authority vested from without the profession. *The medical profession* should insist on the privilege of licensing and regulating its profession with safeguards to protect the public and the individual physician from abuses of privilege. There should be established in jurisdictional governments an independent board or agency or within an established branch of government, an independent division or board, delegating to it full authority to regulate itself and to carry into effect the provisions of an act.[39]

Several articles and publications sparked the debate over board reorganization in the 1970s. Critics accused boards of engaging in anticompetitive and monopolistic behavior, as well as failing to discipline poor practitioners. They proposed "sunsetting" boards out of existence or giving them advisory powers only.[40] The federal government was among those voicing a preference for centralized administration.[41] One federal study concluded: "With administration centralized, occupational groups can continue to be major forces in establishing and enforcing regulatory policies, but through a state agency which can reconcile the interest of the general public with those of the private associations."[42] Other policy experts agreed. William Selden, a leading proponent of reform, urged that states combine all licensing boards into one, with separate committees for each profession.[43] Years later, a task force of the Pew Health Professions Commission partially echoed these sentiments. It recommended that states "consolidate the structure and function of boards around related health professional or health services areas" such as medicine and nursing.[44]

Some states put these recommendations to the test. Virginia established a Board of Health Professions in 1977 to coordinate policy for its twelve licensing boards, including its Board of Medicine.[45] In 1975 New York shifted authority for disciplining physicians accused of incompetence from the Board of Medicine to the Department of Health.[46] Illinois and Nebraska also divested their boards of some disciplinary powers during the 1970s, placing oversight authority in umbrella agencies.[47] Nevertheless, most state agencies, such as New Jersey's Division of Consumer Affairs, went no farther than to furnish medical boards with certain housekeeping or administrative assistance.[48] This situation prompted Stanley Gross to conclude, based on 1980 data, that "the autonomous licensing board is currently alive and well."[49]

Most boards retained policy-making authority, but certain aspects of board reorganization expanded external oversight. Budget and personnel issues were key. Large health departments and other central agencies of state governments often had the power to allocate funds and to hire and fire staff of subordinate agencies or departments. Central agencies that subsumed board operations could indirectly influence medical discipline through budgetary review. Fiscal constraints affected board functions, just as they did those of other state agencies. The amount of money available for medical boards increased following reorganization, but increases were marginal as state governments imposed strict limits on budgets and personnel. According to the Office of the Inspector General for the Department of Health and Human Services, "severe budgetary constraints are precluding boards from adding sufficiently to their corps of investigators and from making investments in computer technology and training that could improve productivity over time."[50] Testifying before a congressional subcommittee in 1990, the executive director of Oregon's medical board remarked:

It hasn't been emphasized enough. Medical boards traditionally were independent up until about 20 years ago, and about a third or 40 percent of the medical boards in this country probably now are part of an umbrella agency. I think, frankly, it has hurt them considerably. It did hurt us until we were able to extricate ourselves from that process in 1983. . . . We believe that it is crucial. Why is it crucial? Because it allows us to do two things. It allows us to go directly to the executive department to argue about our budget. More importantly, if they say, no, and frankly in Oregon most budgetary people do say no, . . . it allows us to go to the legislature directly and argue our case and say, here are the things we feel are necessary to run a good medical board, executive department had said no to these decision packages, and we are appealing those decisions to you.[51]

Just as organized medicine hindered medical discipline, so did state governments. State budgets, rules, and regulations hampered flexibility by tying boards' fate to the vicissitudes of state politics and bureaucratic process. In New York, where state bureaucracy was most entrenched, board performance floundered in the 1970s and 1980s.[52] This was because the elaborate review process established to curtail physician involvement in disciplinary matters created a fragmentary system that delayed board action.[53] According to a member of SHAME, the process for reviewing decisions of the New York board "delays disciplinary recommendations by a year or more, and often reduces doctors' disciplinary actions after they have already gone through an investigation and a formal hearing."[54] To expedite medical discipline, SHAME supported legislation that would end external review of board decisions.

The Quest for Organizational Autonomy

During the 1980s the fight for control of state medical boards entered a new phase as physicians mounted a campaign to secure organizational autonomy. This time the fight was primarily over money. Physicians successfully argued that as long as funds for board operations came from the medical community in the form of licensing fees, physicians should control their allocation.

Enhanced physician interest in medical discipline reflected widespread changes in intraprofessional relations during the 1970s and 1980s. Physicians were not only responding to state involvement in board governance, they were also more receptive to efforts to discipline their colleagues. Changes within medicine included formal review of clinical decisions through use of standardized criteria, conversion to a competitive marketplace that lacked professional constraints on fees and advertising, and the incorporation of management practices from the business community.[55] These changes created cleavages within the medical profession, not as had previously occurred through specialization, but through formalization of professional controls. Formal peer review, for example, created distinctions between those practitioners who set standards and those who did not, as did the incorporation of management practices in hospitals and other medical institutions where the authority of physician-administrators became more extensive and more binding on the rank and file. Finally, increased competition among physicians weakened norms and values that had promoted unity by discouraging internal criticism. Despite the bureaucratization of medical practice, physicians continued to regulate themselves, but they were more active in disciplining their colleagues, whether by reviewing grievances under the auspices of state medical boards and federal peer review organizations or by testifying against one another in lawsuits for malpractice.[56]

The Federation of State Medical Boards assumed a leadership role in the fight for organizational autonomy. Established in 1912, the federation's membership comprised medical boards in all fifty states, the District of Columbia, Puerto Rico, Guam, the Virgin Islands, and twelve of sixteen independent state boards of osteopathic medicine.[57] The federation's major source of revenue came from certain licensing exams that it administered on behalf of its component boards.[58] State takeover of board operations threatened the federation's survival by altering its underlying structure.

Seeking to sustain its membership, the federation promoted the "independent" board. An independent board, the federation said, was one that controlled its own resources and had full authority to regulate the medical profession.[59] In its revised *Guide to the Essentials of a Modern Medical Practice Act* published in 1988, the federation insisted that boards have responsibility for the promulgation of their own rules, the review and investigation of complaints, the discipline of licensees, and the establishment of appropriate fees and charges to support their activities. Because board tasks had become large and complex, the federation recommended that boards employ an executive secretary or director and other staff, including investigators and legal counsel. The federation also encouraged boards to develop consistent standards and to share information with one another.[60]

In promoting an independent board, the federation sought to address problems of legal process, case backlogs, and public accountability. Board staff, including investigators, administrators, and attorneys, became the principal means for resolving complaints. Administrators screened cases; investigators interviewed witnesses; lawyers negotiated consent agreements.

All this preceded formal board action that was collegial in nature. These arrangements expedited case review while insulating board members from legal entanglements. According to board members in Michigan, "a well-established and effective staff structure . . . is essential, partially to handle the everyday Board affairs as well as emergencies that arise. Further, consent agreements—the plea bargains—could and probably should be the status of most cases that reach board agendas."[61] Table 3.1 illustrates the comparative features of the professional, bureaucratic, and federation models of medical discipline.

Just as the federation's model sought to expedite case review, so it also sought to preserve physician control over medical discipline. The federation's guide was quite clear on one point: "Whatever the make-up of the Board, physicians should constitute the majority of the membership."[62] The proposed model superimposed a collegial body, composed mainly of physicians, on top of an administrative structure, composed mainly of bureaucrats. On the professional side of the ledger, board members functioned much as corporate directors, meeting to decide important matters as required by law. Board members formed committees to oversee licensing, investigation, finance, administration, personnel, rules, legislative communications, and public information. On the administrative side of the ledger, boards delegated authority to an executive secretary or director who supervised clerical staff and investigators. The federation's model contemplated the use of lawyers, hearing officers, experts, and consultants, some or all of whom came from other agencies of state government.[63]

Federation leaders, in effect, came close to duplicating the organizational structure of acute-care hospitals in which a managerial hierarchy coexisted with a professional staff. The difference was that physicians themselves comprised the governing body that supervised the administrative staff, giving them operational control. Moreover, the board's operating core consisted of government bureaucrats who performed the daily tasks related to licensure and discipline.

Despite these important features, physician domination of board operations mattered little if outside agencies controlled board funds and personnel. Federation leaders did not want to copy the model for federally sponsored peer review organizations, a source of much dissatisfaction within the medical community.[64] As Schattschneider opined, "the *winners* in intrabusiness strife want to be let alone (they want autonomy)."[65] This is precisely what federation leaders wanted for state medical boards.

Boards would achieve independent status, the federation believed, if states channeled revenues from board activities, such as licensing fees, di-

TABLE 3.1
Comparative Features of Professional, Bureaucratic, and Federation Models

Key features	Professional model	Bureaucratic model	Federation model
De facto control	State medical societies	State government	Autonomous board of directors
Dominant form of decision making	Collegial	Hierarchial	Collegial and hierarchial
Funding source	Shared resources/ limited budget	State general funds	Dedicated funds (licensing fees)
Primary mechanisms for controlling behavior	Self-regulating (professional norms and ethics)	Formal sanctions	Consent orders
Role of boards in policing profession	Bolster hospital medical staffs and professional associations	Agencies of State government	Independent actors
Geographic orientation	Local	State	Regional/national
Confidentiality of meetings and records	Closed meetings; physician/patient privilige; peer review	Open meetings; freedom of information acts	Open or closed hearings; limited access to records

rectly into board operations rather than into state general funds.[66] Dedication of licensing fees to board operations not only would provide boards with resources to manage their own caseloads but would also insulate them from budgetary constraints of umbrella agencies. California was among the first states to adopt this strategy during the 1960s. Its board accumulated $470,000 in licensing fees in fiscal year 1960, which it used to hire fifteen investigators.[67] Many states lagged years, even decades, behind as observers agreed that licensing fees often passed into state general funds before 1980.[68] By the early 1980s the federation's campaign for fiscal autonomy took hold. Thirty-one states allowed their boards to dedicate all or a portion of fees collected to cover operations in 1986; forty states authorized their boards to do so in 1996. Those states that switched to dedicated funding between 1986 and 1996 included Maryland, Massachusetts, New York, Ohio, Rhode Island, South Carolina, Tennessee, Utah, and Vermont.[69]

As shown in table 3.2, increasing budgets are explained in part by the establishment of regular and reliable sources of funds under board control. Although the federation did not publish budgetary information on state medical boards before 1993, and Grad and Marti's study surveyed only eight states in 1976, certain patterns were still discernible. First, those boards that failed to supply budgetary information to the federation in 1993 and 1996 usually obtained their money from state general or departmental funds. These boards included Connecticut, Delaware, the District of Columbia, Hawaii, Illinois, Indiana, Michigan, New York (in 1993), and Wisconsin. Second, most boards that states allowed to cover expenses from licensing fees enjoyed substantial growth in revenues during the 1990s, particularly those boards receiving authorization between 1986 and 1996, such as those in Maryland, Massachusetts, Ohio, Rhode Island, South Carolina, and Tennessee.

Because most boards increased their budgets during the 1980s and 1990s, they were able to hire more staff. As shown in table 3.3, overall staffing of state medical boards increased about 100 percent between 1987 and 1996. Boards with dedicated funds, such as those in California, Maryland, Nevada, and Ohio, significantly added to their staff, but so did some boards that received money from state general or departmental funds, such as those in Georgia and Illinois.

The federation's strategy for organizational autonomy freed physicians from the reins of government. By 1996 the federation classified forty-nine state medical boards as independent; four, including the District of Columbia, as subordinate; nine as semi-autonomous; and five as advisory.[70] Table 3.4 relates the federation's classification of state medical boards for the years 1995–96. According to the federation, a board was "independent" if it exercised all licensing and disciplinary powers; its status did not change if a central agency provided some clerical services. "Semi-autonomous" boards, the federation indicated, rendered final decisions in all important licensing and disciplinary matters, but central state agencies controlled budget, staffing, and investigative functions. "Subordinate" boards, including those in Rhode Island and Tennessee, relied on central agencies to review and implement their decisions. "Advisory" boards, like those in Illinois and Utah, had no decision-making authority.[71] Central agencies in these states assumed all licensing and disciplinary functions.

Although most boards gained independence in the sense that they con-

TABLE 3.2

Operating Budgets of State Medical Boards, 1976, 1993, and 1996
(in dollars)

State	1976	1993	1996
Alabama			1,936,790
Alaska		235,000	268,000
Arizona	600,000	2,226,900	2,276,900
Arkansas			850,548
California	5,800,000	24,400,000	29,670,000
Colorado		1,500,000	1,500,000
Connecticut			
Delaware			
District of Columbia			
Florida			10,000,000
Georgia		819,934	819,934
Hawaii			
Idaho		450,000	450,000
Illinois			
Indiana			
Iowa			1,041,000
Kansas			1,467,608
Kentucky		740,000	1,044,000
Louisiana		1,890,000	1,838,000
Maine		455,000	720,000
Maryland	9,000	3,246,083	5,750,083
Massachusetts		1,685,000	2,900,000
Michigan	379,985		
Minnesota		2,488,000	2,488,000
Mississippi	130,000	663,000	726,201
Missouri			1,703,073
Montana		333,493	333,493
Nebraska			361,875
Nevada		630,600	630,600
New Hampshire		203,328	292,000
New Jersey		3,500,000	5,300,000
New Mexico		530,000	530,000
New York	450,000		
North Carolina		2,036,246	2,036,246
North Dakota		226,842	226,842

State	1976	1993	1996
Ohio		2,953,002	4,676,984
Oklahoma		1,200,000	1,685,887
Oregon		1,852,732	2,205,193
Pennsylvania	150,000		2,348,000
Rhode Island			1,177,065
South Carolina	235,557		1,258,053
South Dakota			
Tennessee			930,275
Texas		3,473,861	4,100,000
Utah			
Vermont		307,000	307,000
Virginia			2,958,480
Washington		6,400,000	6,400,000
West Virginia		850,000	850,000
Wisconsin			
Wyoming		233,808	240,351

Source: Data from Grad and Marti, *Physicians' Licensure and Discipline,* 431. Federation of State Medical Boards, *Exchange* (1992–93): 23, (1995–96): 23.

Note: For comparative purposes, only allopathic medical boards for each of the fifty states and the District of Columbia are included.

trolled their internal operations, they required assistance from outside agencies and their personnel to perform certain disciplinary functions. When boards sought legal advice, for instance, they usually secured it from the office of the state attorney general.[72] When boards engaged hearing officers to preside over hearings and prepare written findings for board ratification, they often turned to an outside agency.[73]

Employing lawyers, hearing officers, investigators, and administrative personnel to perform essential functions transformed boards as disciplinary bodies. Physicians had always been in the forefront in managing, investigating, and adjudicating board cases. Now physicians shared responsibility with nonphysicians and government bureaucrats. Board members began to distance themselves from the day-to-day operations. Executive directors, who were often nonphysicians, assumed control over routine matters. Boards still acted as collegial bodies in rendering final decisions, but their underlying structure became bureaucratic. Resolving complaints against physicians involved many steps, any one of which could affect the outcome. Casting a wary eye on these developments, some board members observed that "one

TABLE 3.3

Number of Full-Time, Part-Time, and Temporary/Seasonal Staff Employed by or Assigned to the State Medical Boards, 1976, 1987, and 1996

State	1976	1987	1996
Alabama		11	17
Alaska			3.5
Arizona	6	28	40
Arkansas		4	6
California	40	170	318
Colorado		7	12
Connecticut			5
Delaware			4
District of Columbia		7	5
Florida		12	31.5
Georgia		11	20
Hawaii		1.5	5
Idaho		4	5
Illinois			76
Indiana			5
Iowa		14	18
Kansas		14	29
Kentucky		15	16
Louisiana		15	38
Maine		4	5
Maryland	2	10	53
Massachusetts		58	52
Michigan			
Minnesota		14	29
Mississippi	4	8	14
Missouri		23	27
Nebraska		5	7
Nevada		4	31
New Hampshire		2	4
New Jersey		17	30
New Mexico		1.5	11
New York		2	4
North Carolina		10	23
North Dakota		3	4

State	1976	1987	1996
Ohio		30	77
Oklahoma		12	27
Oregon		16.5	29
Pennsylvania	2	1	30
Rhode Island		5	8
South Carolina	5	15	19
South Dakota		1	2
Tennessee		6	21
Texas		57	54
Utah			5
Vermont		0.5	7
Virginia		12	20
Washington		7	33
West Virginia		6	12
Wisconsin		2.5	2.5
Total	59*	646.5*	1294.5*

Source: Data from Grad and Marti, *Physicians' Licensure and Discipline,* 431; Federation of State Medical Boards, *Exchange* (1987): 15, (1995–96): 16–17.

Note: For comparative purposes, only allopathic medical boards for each of the fifty states and the District of Columbia are included.

*Based solely on available information.

of the great disadvantages of staff determining the outcome of allegations . . . is the marked increased capacity for the regulatory bureaucracy to develop and entrench its own beliefs, the skillful maneuvering of the board, the information limits in the name of efficiency, and the somewhat callous regard to outcomes so long as outcomes occur with some dispatch."[74]

Conclusion

From about the 1970s to the 1990s, most state medical boards made the transition from small-scale operations to bureaucratic organizations that could manage large and growing caseloads. For many boards, this transition was difficult. Physicians who feared government control of the disciplinary process clung to a professional model of decision making that stressed informality, collegiality, and confidentiality. The professional model, inadequate for the task at hand, failed to accommodate changing political, social, and economic conditions that stressed professional accountability. The bureaucratic model was more in tune with the times. A more formal structure

TABLE 3.4
Relationship of State Medical Boards to Agencies of
State Government

Board	Status	Agency Relationship
Alabama	Independent	Board is totally independent
Alaska	Seim-autonomous	Most services are provided by Division of Occupational Licensing, Department of Commerce and Economic Development
Arizona		
M	Independent	Some services are provided by the Department of Administration
O	Independent	Some services are provided by other state agencies
Arkansas	Independent	Some services are provided by other state agencies
California		
M	Independent	Some services are provided by Department of Consumer Affairs
O	Independent	Some services are provided by other state agencies
Colorado	Independent	Most services are provided by Department of Consumer Affairs
Connecticut	Subordinate	Department of Public Health and Addiction Services handles most administrative matters and has final authority on most substantial issues except that board adjudicates disciplinary cases
Delaware	Independent	Most services are provided by Department of Administrative Services, Division of Professional Regulation
District of Columbia	Subordinate	Within Department of Consumer and Regulatory Affairs
Florida		
M	Semi-autonomous	Within Agency for Health Care Administration
O	Semi-autonomous	Within Agency for Health Care Administration
Georgia	Independent	Administrative support provided by office of the Secretary of State

Board	Status	Agency Relationship
Guam	Independent	Most services are provided by Department of Public Health and Social Services
Hawaii	Independent	Most services are provided by Department of Commerce and Consumer Affairs
Idaho	Independent	(No further information reported by board)
Illinois	Advisory	Department of Professional Regulation has final authority on licensure and disciplinary functions
Indiana	Independent	Most services are provided by Health Professions Bureau
Iowa	Independent	Budget submitted through Health Department
Kansas	Independent	Some services are provided by Department of Administration
Kentucky	Independent	Some services are provided by Cabinet for Human Resources and Office of Attorney General
Louisiana	Independent	Within the Department of Health and Hospitals
Maine		
M	Independent	Affiliated for administrative support and liaison with chief executive/legislature with Department of Professional and Financial Regulation
O	Independent	Affiliated for administrative support and liaison with chief executive/legislature with Department of Professional and Financial Regulation
Maryland	Semi-autonomous	Within the Department of Health and Mental Hygiene
Massachusetts	Semi-autonomous	Within Office of Consumer Affairs and Business Regulation
Michigan		
M	Independent	Most services are provided by Department of Commerce, Office of Health Services
O	Independent	Most services are provided by Department of Commerce, Office of Health Services
Minnesota	Independent	Some services are provided by other state agencies

TABLE 3.4 (continued)

Board	Status	Agency Relationship
Mississippi	Independent	(No further information reported by board)
Missouri	Independent	Some services are provided by Division of Professional Registration
Montana	Independent	Most services are provided by Department of Commerce
Nebraska	Subordinate	Department of Health handles most administrative matters; Director of Health has final authority on most substantial issues and all disciplinary actions
Nevada		
M	Independent	(No further information reported by board)
O	Independent	(No further information reported by board)
New Hampshire	Independent	(No further information reported by board)
New Jersey	Independent	Some services provided by Division of Consumer Affairs
New Mexico		
M	Independent	Administratively aligned through Department of Financial and Professional Regulation
O	Independent	Administratively attached to Department of Regulation and Licensing
New York	Advisory	New York State Board of Regents has final authority on licensure, New York State Department of Health, Board of Professional Medical Conduct
North Carolina	Independent	(No further information reported by board)
North Dakota	Independent	Board is totally independent
Ohio	Independent	(No further information reported by board)
Oklahoma		
M	Independent	Autonomous board; nonappropriated funds; all services provided by board
O	Independent	Not applicable
Oregon	Independent	Executive Department of the State of Oregon
Pennsylvania		
M	Independent	Most services are provided by Department of State, Bureau of Professional and Occupational Affairs

Board	Status	Agency Relationship
O	Independent	Most services are provided by Department of State, Bureau of Professional and Occupational Affairs
Puerto Rico	Independent	(No further information reported by board)
Rhode Island	Semi-autonomous	Department of Health handles most administrative matters and has final authority on most substantial issues except board licensing and adjudication of disciplinary cases
South Carolina	Independent	Department of Labor, Licensing, and Regulation handles most administrative matters
South Dakota	Independent	Department of Commerce and Regulation
Tennessee		
M	Subordinate	Department of Health and Environment, Division of Health-Related Boards handles most administrative matters
O	Subordinate	Department of Health and Environment, Division of Health-Related Boards handles most administrative matters
Texas	Independent	Board is totally independent
Utah		
M	Advisory	Division of Occupational and Professional Licensing has final authority on disciplinary functions
O	Advisory	Division of Occupational and Professional Licensing has final authority on disciplinary functions
Vermont		
M	Independent	Some services are provided by Office of the Secretary of State, Office of Professional Regulation
O	Independent	Services are provided by Office of the Secretary of State, Office of Professional Regulation
Virginia	Semi-autonomous	Department of Health Professions handles most administrative matters and has final authority on budget and hiring. Board has final authority on regulations and disciplinary decisions.
Virgin Islands	Advisory	Department of Health

TABLE 3.4 (continued)

Board	Status	Agency Relationship
Washington		
M	Semi-autonomous	Within the Department of Licensing
O	Semi-autonomous	Department of Health handles most administrative matters
West Virginia		
M	Independent	(No further information reported by board)
O	Independent	None
Wisconsin	Independent	Within the Department of Regulation and Licensing
Wyoming	Independent	Some services are provided by Department of Administration and Fiscal Control

Source: Federation of State Medical Boards, *Exchange* (1995–96): 2–3.

Key: M = medical; O = osteopathic. Independent = 49; subordinate = 5; semi-autonomous = 9; advisory = 5.

promised greater uniformity, continuity, and standardization of performance, features required if boards were to satisfy public expectations. Reconciling the two models pitted professional and public interests or, as Schattschneider would say, the conflicting tendencies toward the privatization and the socialization of conflict. Consumers and the media championed state governments; physicians still looked to their state and local medical societies.

Building a modern state medical board required money and resources. State governments were reluctant to provide them absent political control. Having much to lose if central agencies of state government gained the upper hand, the Federation of State Medical Boards promoted the concept of an independent board. Although few states divested their boards of policy-making authority in the 1970s, many influenced board operations by controlling budgets and personnel. Seeking a reliable source of funds for hiring their own staff, boards lobbied state legislatures in the 1980s and 1990s to channel licensing fees directly into board coffers rather than into state general funds. Most succeeded. By 1996 thirty-seven out of fifty-one state medical boards were independent in the sense that they exercised all licensing and disciplinary powers and controlled their own resources. Of the remaining fourteen, several enjoyed dedicated funding or experienced increased staffing as states poured funds into medical discipline.

Public pressure mounted for improved performance in the wake of board reorganizations and increased resources. Raw numbers would not suffice; boards also had to tackle substantive complaints that federal agencies, state governments, consumer groups, and the press recognized as important. These included cases involving physician drug abuse, sexual misconduct, and professional incompetence. Responding to external pressures, boards moved from a professional model of decision making that stressed informality, collegiality, and confidentiality to one that emphasized legal process, case management, and public accountability. Physicians, in effect, formed their own bureaucracy to avoid control by another. Having secured their authority over board operations, physicians now had to discipline their fellow colleagues. The price of power in the 1980s and 1990s was increased accountability. Boards had to regulate the profession efficiently and effectively if they were to avoid further adverse scrutiny.

CHAPTER FOUR

Balancing Public and Professional Concerns

Before the 1980s most boards lacked the institutional capacity to survive on their own in a pluralist environment. Managing a complex and growing caseload was only part of the problem. The real test was in moderating the conflicting tendencies toward the privatization and the socialization of conflict. Although physicians still controlled medical discipline following attempts by states to centralize board operations, the public was no longer excluded. Government intervention in medical discipline widened the scope of conflict, forcing boards to devise means for controlling it. Board members who favored education and rehabilitation of physicians yet recognized the need for public protection struggled to accommodate public and professional concerns.

As we have seen, the aggregate number of disciplinary actions against licensed physicians substantially increased once boards altered their mission and developed the capacity to pursue poor practitioners on their own. But this was only a part of the story. Aggregate numbers failed to reflect the shifting direction of state medical board prosecutions. The types of cases that boards prosecuted was undergoing a fundamental transformation as depicted in figure 4.1. In particular, disciplinary actions against physicians for substandard care, incompetence, or negligence jumped from seven during the period 1963–67 to 1,677 during the period 1986–96.[1]

As long as physicians were the dominant force in health care, organized medicine set the agenda. The types of cases that boards prosecuted involved doctors who ventured outside the professional mainstream—abortionists, drug addicts, and "unorthodox" providers. In many instances, law enforcement agencies or state medical societies had already investigated these physicians for their misbehavior. Boards had neither the ability nor the inclination to pursue physicians for malpractice or unprofessional conduct on their own. These matters were best left to professional associations and medical staff of hospitals.

Having obtained more money and resources, boards received pressure from the media, consumers, insurers, government bureaucrats, and politicians to alter the agenda. Boards revoked licenses for sexual misconduct because consumers targeted patient abuse. Boards focused on incompetent practitioners because states linked medical malpractice with lack of physician discipline. Boards prosecuted physicians for fraud because federal officials feared rising costs.

More aggressive boards on behalf of consumers and other interests alarmed organized medicine. Different philosophies prevailed in the professional and law-enforcement communities concerning proper review and punishment of physicians guilty of misconduct or incompetence. Organized medicine preferred confidential peer review and rehabilitation of offenders; consumers and government officials sought public accountability and punitive action. Boards were caught in the middle. Their new role required them to protect the public, not the profession. Yet, most board members were physicians. They had the delicate task of balancing the interests of government and society with those of their calling.

Perceiving a threat to their interests, professional associations sought to curtail board initiatives. They established committees to monitor board operations and created programs that could serve as alternatives to disciplinary action. At the heart of these efforts were disagreements over who should take the lead in regulating professional misconduct and how it should be accomplished. Organized medicine sought to keep conflict private. Consumers used media and government agencies to widen its scope. The struggle of state medical boards for organizational autonomy reflected the need to reconcile these polar interests.

Three confrontations between boards and professional associations in the late 1980s and early 1990s over the investigation and prosecution of physicians for drug and alcohol abuse, sexual misconduct, and incompetence are examined below in a case study format. These were among the most controversial issues that boards faced because of their implications for physicians and their patients. In each instance, the AMA and the Federation of State Medical Boards carefully reviewed the problem and issued one or more statements of policy that guided actions of their component organizations.[2]

The first case study, involving drug and alcohol abuse among physicians, gained notoriety in the 1970s when researchers revealed the widespread nature of the problem and boards took action to control it. State medical societies responded with the formation of impaired physicians programs that emphasized confidentiality and rehabilitation of substance abusers. The refusal of such programs to share the names of impaired physicians with state medical boards led to confrontations in several states over public access and monitoring. Perhaps the most significant confrontation

FIGURE 4.1

Comparison of reasons for disciplinary actions, 1963–1967 and 1986–1996.

Source: Data from Derbyshire, *Medical Licensure and Discipline,* 78; Wolfe et al., *Questionable Doctors* (1996), 23.

*Not applicable to corresponding time frame.

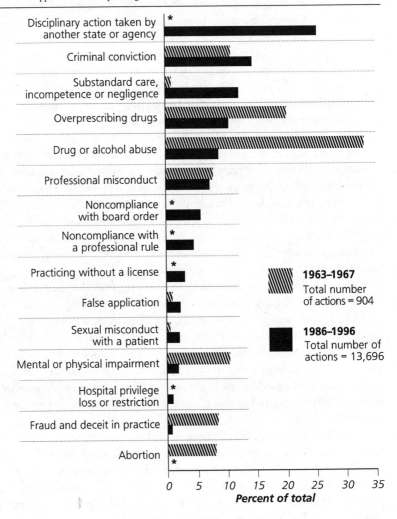

occurred in New Jersey where a government investigation spawned media interest and court litigation that pitted the state medical board against the state medical society.

Few topics stirred more controversy than sexual exploitation of patients by physicians, the subject of the second case study. Some called it the regulatory issue of the 1990s.[3] Although impaired physicians found shelter in rehabilitation programs, those guilty of sexually exploiting their patients rarely did. Absent a means for controlling sexual offenders, state boards either revoked physicians' licenses or faced public ridicule. Even so, many avoided the problem through delay or other means. Dissatisfied with the official response, consumers pressured lawmakers to overhaul state boards and pass legislation making sexual misconduct by physicians a crime.[4] Consumer activism served as a wake-up call for the medical community. Foot-dragging by physicians only made things worse. The media sensed a good story and went after it with vigor, particularly in Massachusetts, where the *Boston Globe* ran a series of articles highlighting the lack of board action.[5] Subsequent efforts by the Massachusetts board to correct the situation inflamed the medical community, leading to court challenges and legislative initiatives.

The subject of the third case study is physician incompetence. Attempts to discipline physicians for incompetence had their roots in the medical malpractice crises of the 1970s and 1980s. Despite the tenuous linkage between malpractice and incompetence, states passed laws that required health-care providers and entities to report medical malpractice to state medical boards. Inundated with these complaints, some boards sought to resolve them through use of medical consultants, nurses, advisory committees, and peer review organizations of hospitals and the federal government.[6] Maryland was unique in that its board engaged state and local medical societies to conduct peer review. When investigations of physicians for incompetence floundered in Maryland, the *Washington Post* attacked the relationship between the state medical board and the state medical society, claiming that the board had become "a creature of the medical establishment."[7]

These three case studies illustrate the problems that boards encountered in reconciling the attributes of the professional and bureaucratic models of decision making. Gaining the resources and expertise to determine professional misconduct, formulate standards for prosecution, fashion options for education and rehabilitation, and assess compliance with board orders was a political process that involved more than simply accumulating money and staff. For physicians to retain control, they needed to institutionalize private means of enforcement. Programs that stressed rehabilitation, education, and peer review counterbalanced the more formal and punitive aspects of medical discipline.

Rehabilitating the Impaired Physician

Physician impairment refers to "the inability to practice medicine with reasonable skill and safety because of physical or mental illness."[8] Most instances of physician impairment concern substance abuse and addiction. The remainder involve loss of cognitive, motor, or perceptive skills unrelated to chemical dependency.[9] Estimates of drug and alcohol addiction in the physician population range from 10 to 15 percent.[10] Studies show that the risk of addiction is higher and detection is more difficult among doctors than in most other groups. Reasons include job stress, easy access to mood-altering drugs, the ability to self-prescribe, and inadequate oversight within the medical community.[11]

In the 1950s state boards began to explore mechanisms for rehabilitating impaired physicians. California led the way. Rather than revoke licenses of impaired physicians outright, California's board placed substance abusers on probation after taking away their right to prescribe dangerous drugs. The terms of probation often included psychiatric supervision and frequent monitoring of progress. Using this approach, California placed 130 physicians on probation for drug addiction between 1948 and 1957, revoking only eight licenses during that period.[12]

Although several states followed California's lead, medical practice acts hampered their efforts by predicating disciplinary action on proof of impaired clinical judgment or actual injury to a patient.[13] Beginning with Florida in 1969, two-thirds of the states passed "sick doctor statutes" over the next ten years making it easier for boards to intervene in cases of physician impairment. These laws gave boards the authority to conduct physical or mental examinations of physicians suspected of abusing drugs or alcohol. Most laws guaranteed confidentiality of examination results and provided immunity protection from civil lawsuits for those supplying information on impaired physicians.[14]

Sick doctor statutes had the backing of organized medicine.[15] Indeed, the AMA drafted the model legislation enacted in many states.[16] Yet enhanced board activity became a growing source of concern to the medical profession. A study of Oregon physicians conducted between 1976 and 1977 indicated that the suicide rate among physicians on probation or under state board investigation was unusually high.[17] Political and consumer pressures on boards to increase discipline threatened efforts to rehabilitate impaired physicians. The executive director of Alabama's medical association cautioned that "if organized medicine does not take a leadership role in [physician impairment], someone else will: the licensing boards, plaintiff attorneys, or the state legislatures. Their impetus definitely will be punitive rather than treatment oriented."[18] These fears were widespread within the medical community.[19]

Responding to enforcement initiatives of state boards, state medical societies began forming impaired physician committees in the 1970s. Official endorsement for these committees occurred in 1972 when the AMA's Council on Mental Health reported several studies documenting the prevalence of drug and alcohol abuse among physicians and efforts by state medical boards to address it. Noting that only seven state societies had committees on physician impairment, the council called on other societies to become active. Punitive action in the form of license revocation or suspension, the council suggested, did not further early detection and rehabilitation. Self-policing was necessary to protect the public.[20]

Organized medicine sought to minimize board involvement in these cases. By 1984 medical societies in all fifty states had established their own programs to deal with physician impairment.[21] These programs, known as impaired physicians programs or IPPs, stressed the need for absolute confidentiality and rehabilitation of substance abusers.[22] Few IPPs had any formal relationship with state government, and most refused to share names of impaired physicians with their state board counterparts. Such programs often became advocates for physicians in matters affecting licensure, malpractice insurance, and hospital privileges.[23] In some states, relationships between boards and IPPs were cooperative; in others, they were confrontational.[24] Problems arose in attempting to reconcile the public interest with those of impaired physicians.

Professional associations marshaled support for IPPs in several ways. Medical directors of IPPs kept statistics to demonstrate their success in rehabilitating impaired physicians. They published numerous articles in medical journals documenting their results.[25] Although relatively small numbers of physicians entered IPPs, program directors claimed that they had achieved a rehabilitation rate of about 90 percent.[26]

The high rate of success in rehabilitating impaired physicians called attention to certain attributes of IPPs. These included treatment and monitoring, not discipline, and absolute confidentiality, not public disclosure. Punitive measures, advocates claimed, discouraged reporting and jeopardized rehabilitation. Physicians who were in treatment and under close supervision, they said, could continue to practice medicine safely and effectively despite their addiction. In states where laws mandated the reporting of impaired physicians to state boards, referrals actually declined.[27] Professional associations asserted that self-regulation not only aided the impaired physician but also enhanced public protection. Because physicians and others in the medical community were more likely to report impaired physicians to a confidential treatment program than to a state board, such programs increased oversight. Because program administrators conducted studies showing that physicians continued to practice safely under program auspices, public exposure and discipline were counterproductive.[28]

Emboldened by their initial success, advocates of self-regulation warned professional societies against collaborating with state boards. Edward Carden, a member of the AMA's National Advisory Committee on Impaired Physicians, claimed that "a state bureaucratic process" was "less effective and more expensive" in regulating physician impairment than were programs run exclusively by state medical societies: "Perhaps it's as simple as America's traditional and healthy lack of trust in the power of bureaucracies."[29] G. Douglas Talbott, director of the Impaired Physicians Program for the Medical Association of Georgia, agreed. He asserted that joint programs between boards and state medical societies were "ineffective" because they "tend[ed] to become punitive rather than advocatory in nature."[30]

The arguments that organized medicine raised in favor of a confidential, nondisciplinary approach were persuasive. During the mid-1980s state boards reexamined their role in disciplining physicians for substance abuse. IPPs, some board administrators observed, provided a reasonable alternative to disciplinary action in many instances.[31] Still, the dilemma remained for boards seeking to balance public and professional concerns. Because most IPPs were physician-sponsored organizations, they lacked public accountability. Many feared that, if left on their own, IPPs would fail to monitor adequately impaired physicians, endangering patient safety. In New Jersey a controversy erupted between the state board and the medical society that underscored these concerns.

The New Jersey Experience

Like many other state medical societies, the Medical Society of New Jersey (MSNJ) established an impaired physicians committee in the late 1970s and replaced it with an IPP in the 1980s. MSNJ was the first, however, to hire a full-time medical director, David Canavan, in 1982. Canavan had almost thirty years' experience in the field of chemical dependency. With the help of his assistant director, a Roman Catholic priest named Edward Reading, Canavan made New Jersey's program a model for the rest of the country (*New York Times,* 13 Mar. 1987). According to the director of Georgia's program, Canavan established "a superb patient recovery record augmented by excellent case record documentation."[32] Programs in other states, including those in Florida, New York, Tennessee, and Pennsylvania, followed New Jersey's lead.

Canavan's success attracted the attention of state officials. New Jersey's Board of Medical Examiners had no access to the names of physicians entering Canavan's program. As was the case before MSNJ established an IPP, the flow of information to the state board "remained negligible."[33] Concerned about the role of MSNJ in regulating impaired physicians, the New Jersey State Commission of Investigation (SCI) began to examine Canavan's practices and procedures.

Created in 1968 as a weapon against organized crime and political corruption in New Jersey, SCI began to branch out in the 1980s.[34] One of the SCI commissioners, James R. Zazzali, favored tougher laws on physician incompetence. As attorney general of New Jersey in 1981, Zazzali pursued legislation requiring all health-care professionals to report impaired and incompetent physicians to the state board. After his legislation failed to pass, Zazzali sought to build a record that established the need for mandatory reporting laws in New Jersey.

The SCI's report, released in 1987, caused a stir in New Jersey's medical community. Although critical of hospitals, insurance companies, and state agencies for inadequately monitoring and reporting physician incompetence, SCI reserved its harshest criticism for MSNJ's IPP. Based on voluminous testimony and documentation, the report contained numerous instances where the program had failed to alert public authorities about physicians who SCI believed were a threat to patient safety.

The SCI report related cases where anesthesiologists, neurosurgeons, and other physicians who were substance abusers operated on patients and prescribed drugs, despite their failure to comply with the conditions for participation in the IPP. In several of these cases, SCI claimed, the state board was never notified and given the opportunity to take disciplinary action. The authors of the report asserted that

> the degree to which the [program] concentrates on rescuing the careers of fallen physicians at the potentially deadly expense of patient safety is particularly demonstrated by the program's mothering reaction to uncooperative clients. Far too many impaired physicians who should be reported to the [board] for disciplinary action because they cannot or refuse to complete ther-

apy are, instead, often permitted to resume their practices, including surgery and other perilous tasks, while still chemically addicted or otherwise incompetent.[35]

Physicians, hospital administrators, and program directors, SCI maintained, engaged in a "conspiracy of silence" to deter reporting of impaired physicians to the state board. The IPP created the impression, SCI suggested, that it was the legal authority for receiving complaints about physicians under state law. When there was cause for the IPP to report to the board, referrals had to survive a "bureaucratic obstacle course." First, the program director, Canavan, had to recommend referral to the state board. Next, the impaired physicians committee of MSNJ had to affirm Canavan's decision. Finally, the Board of Trustees of MSNJ had to concur.[36]

Based on its findings, SCI concluded that legislation was needed to improve identification of impaired physicians. Laws that encouraged physicians to report voluntarily by exempting them from liability if they provided information to the state board were not enough. It recommended legislation compelling physicians, health-care facilities, and treatment programs to report to the state board. The state board, it submitted, should act as a "clearinghouse" for all information on impaired physicians in New Jersey. To that end, the SCI recommended that the state board employ a full-time medical director and obtain other resources sufficient to manage cases involving impaired physicians.[37]

MSNJ did not respond publicly to the statements contained in the SCI report. Rather than wage a public relations campaign in the media, MSNJ attacked SCI's recommendations in the state legislature.[38] No one could mistake the anger of its members over SCI's charges. The AMA's Carden called the report a "hatchet job." He claimed that SCI commissioners carefully selected 20 of 380 cases under program auspices and then "consciously misinterpreted and misrepresented" their facts to "create a 'public outcry' for mandatory reporting to the State Board."[39] Herbert Stern, a former federal judge and United States Attorney for New Jersey, added his voice as MSNJ's lawyer. The idea of a "conspiracy of silence," he said, was "outrageous" and a "cheap shot at doctors" (*New York Times*, 20 Dec. 1987).

The controversy involving MSNJ and the state board over monitoring of impaired physicians continued and even intensified in the wake of the SCI report. In 1989 New Jersey enacted legislation requiring that physicians report to the board colleagues who they believed presented a danger to their patients because of gross incompetence or impairment.[40] As one commentator suggested, "now, a practitioner's duty to report an impaired or incompetent colleague is not simply grounded in medical ethics, but in statutory law."[41]

If reformers thought mandatory reporting laws would increase the likelihood that physicians would report their impaired colleagues, they were mistaken. Only five doctors filed reports with the board in the four years following passage of the legislation (*Record*, 21 Dec. 1994). By contrast, physicians themselves accounted for 70 percent of all referrals to the IPP (*Record*, 19 Dec. 1994). The total number of cases referred to the IPP from 1982 to 1993 exceeded eight hundred.

Frustrated with the lack of reporting, state authorities pursued other means of obtaining information about impaired physicians. Like many states, New Jersey required physicians to renew their licenses every two years. In 1991 the state board included the following questions, among others, on its license renewal application:

—Are you now or have you been dependent on alcohol or drugs?

—Are you now or have you been in treatment for alcohol or drug abuse?

—Have you been terminated or granted a leave of absence by a hospital, health care facility, HMO, or any employer for reasons that related to any drug or alcohol use or abuse?

The information requested covered a ten-year period from July 1, 1981 to June 30, 1991.[42] Many other states asked similar questions of their applicants.[43]

Soon after the board mailed the renewal application to licensees, MSNJ sued the board in state court, claiming that the questions violated New Jersey law. The New Jersey Supreme Court ruled in favor of the board,[44] but MSNJ was not finished. In 1993 MSNJ sued the board in federal court alleging that the questions violated Title II of the Americans with Disabilities Act (ADA). Title II of the ADA prohibits a public entity, such as a state licensing board, from discriminating against a "qualified individual with a disability." These questions, MSNJ maintained, improperly targeted doctors, many of whom were qualified to practice medicine, simply on the basis of their disability.

This time, the outcome was different. The U.S. Department of Justice filed an *amicus* brief with the court supporting MSNJ's position. The department claimed that the questions improperly focused on an applicant's status as a person with a disability. The state board had the right to ensure that physicians practiced medicine safely and competently, but it had gone too far. After all, the board had other means of obtaining information on impaired physicians, including patient complaints, malpractice suits, and physician reporting of impaired colleagues. New Jersey's recent mandatory reporting law, the department asserted, "will provide additional information to the Board and will further make the Board's improper inquiries unnecessary."[45]

Although the federal court refused to grant a preliminary injunction in MSNJ's favor, it issued a strongly worded opinion making clear its future intentions. These questions, the court believed, were being used improperly to "screen" physicians for further investigation. Reciting the Justice Department's brief, the court recommended that the board obtain its information from other sources, including reports from doctors about their impaired colleagues.[46]

Following the court's ruling, the board revised the relicensure questions,[47] as did boards in most other states. Questions seeking information on impaired physicians now stated, "Has the use of drugs and/or alcohol resulted in an impairment of your ability to practice your profession?"[48] Designed to accommodate federal law, questions framed in this manner were clearly impractical for eliciting information on impaired physicians. Physicians were no more likely to answer affirmatively to such questions than they were to report impaired colleagues to the board under New Jersey's mandatory reporting law.

The rift between the New Jersey board and MSNJ over the direction and control of the IPP received a great deal of public attention because of the SCI report and the ADA litigation. Although not as pronounced, disputes in other states arose when boards competed with medical societies for control of IPPs.[49] As the ADA litigation in New Jersey indicated, courts were sometimes drawn into the conflict.

Asking courts to protect the confidentiality of physicians who were substance abusers placed physicians and consumers in opposing camps. Judges struggled to balance doctors' right to privacy against consumers' right to know.[50] Licensing boards seeking treatment records faced a welter of federal and state laws prohibiting the disclosure of medical records except in special circumstances.[51] Substance abuse programs that received federal assistance could not even divulge treatment records to law enforcement agencies, including those exercising subpoena powers under state law.[52] Moreover, courts recognized that impaired physicians had a constitutional right to privacy that prevented boards from obtaining treatment records in the absence of a compelling state interest.[53] Boards had to show that no other means existed for obtaining the requested information.[54]

Because securing drug and alcohol treatment records was difficult, IPPs had the upper hand. The enactment of the ADA in 1990 further strengthened their position. The best way for boards to monitor impaired physicians was through a cooperative arrangement with IPPs. As it turned out, IPPs needed boards almost as much as boards needed them. IPPs used boards as leverage to coerce physicians to enter programs and remain in treatment.[55] Canavan and other program directors required impaired physicians to sign contracts agreeing to stay in treatment and abide by program parameters. Physicians who breached the terms of their contracts faced expulsion from the IPP and subsequent disciplinary action, with boards acting as the disciplinarians.

Most IPPs also required some form of outside assistance to fund their operations. For example, New Jersey's IPP increased its budget from $154,000 to $285,000 in its first five years of operation in order to satisfy demand for its services. The IPP could employ a full-time medical director and other staff because malpractice insurance carriers in New Jersey provided financial support.[56] In states where financial support from outside sources was lacking, medical societies had to increase dues anywhere from 10 to 20 percent to adequately staff their programs. Consequently, many IPPs relied on state governments for financial assistance. New York provided grants totaling $800,000 during the mid-1980s.[57] Several states, including Florida, Kentucky, North Carolina, Washington, and Maryland, allocated a portion of license fees to support IPPs.[58] Where state funds were unavailable, IPPs turned to insurance carriers, HMOs, hospitals, and medical societies for help.[59]

By 1995 several IPPs had written agreements with boards outlining the criteria for referral between the two entities. The Federation of State Medical Boards helped to formulate and standardize the terms of the relationship. It recommended that boards execute a formal contract with the IPP that stressed "open lines of communication" and recognized the board's "mission to protect the public."[60] Despite their historical differences, the IPP in New Jersey reached agreement with the state board in 1995 to have an independent entity review and monitor its operations.[61]

Physician impairment is a complex problem requiring disciplinary bodies to craft solutions that balanced the interests of the public and the medical profession. Government-based initiatives backfired because they failed to gain the trust of the medical community. State laws requiring physicians to report their impaired colleagues met an almost total lack of compliance. Relationships between boards and IPPs deteriorated. Government coercion, in this instance, was an inadequate substitute for voluntary self-regulation.

By the same token, physicians failed to regulate themselves in the absence of government coercion. Prospects for rehabilitating impaired physicians were not the only incentives driving the formation of IPPs. Medical societies established IPPs because state boards became more active in disciplining impaired physicians during the 1970s and 1980s. Physicians, to preserve their autonomy, had to develop practical alternatives to government regulation that protected the public as well as members of the profession. IPPs succeeded where grievance committees failed since they were not hobbled by antitrust actions. But as the next case study reveals, some problems were not amenable to self-regulation. Intense consumer and media involvement signaled that only public discipline would suffice. In such instances, state medical boards and state medical societies had few alternatives. Boards and societies ignored such matters at their peril.

Disciplining Physicians Who Sexually Exploit Their Patients

Medical ethicists agree that sexual contact or sexual relations between physicians and their patients is unethical.[62] The traditional role that doctors assume in caring for their patients precludes action that might harm them. From the profession's earliest times, sex with patients qualified as harmful activity. The Hippocratic Oath includes the following prohibition against sexual relations: "I will come for the benefit of the sick, remaining free of all intentional injustice, of all mischief and in particular of sexual relations with both male and female persons."[63]

The medical profession also recognizes that the relationship between physicians and their patients is unequal.[64] Doctors have superior knowledge and expertise; and, in most instances, their patients come to them in a weakened condition due to physical or mental illness. Physicians are not supposed to take advantage of their patients' vulnerability.[65] Because of their dominant position in the relationship, physicians are fiduciaries.[66] Patients entrust them with their care, and physicians have a responsibility to safeguard their patients' trust. Courts often find that sex with a patient constitutes a breach of the physician's fiduciary duty.[67]

Experts have difficulty determining how often sexual exploitation occurs because so much goes unreported.[68] According to one study, 7.1 percent of male psychiatrists and 3.1 percent of female psychiatrists admitted to sexual contact with their patients.[69] In another study, nearly two-thirds of psychiatrists surveyed reported that they had treated patients who had sexual contact with a former therapist, most often another psychiatrist.[70] Although much of the literature on the subject concerns psychiatry, sexual misconduct is not confined to any particular specialty within the field of medicine.[71] Studies show that among nonpsychiatric physicians, 10 percent of male physicians and 4 percent of female physicians report sexual contact with their patients.[72]

Sexual contact between physicians and their patients occurs in a variety of ways and in a variety of settings. In most instances, the physician is male and the patient is female.[73] Examples of sexual contact during treatment range from therapeutic deception to sexual assault. Therapeutic deception refers to claims by physicians that sexual contact is part of the treatment procedure. Sexual assault encompasses rape or fondling of incompetent or unconscious patients. It also includes improper physical examinations of patients.[74] In its 1996 *Report on Sexual Boundary Issues,* an Ad Hoc Committee of the Federation of State Medical Boards distinguished between "sexual violation" and "sexual impropriety." Sexual violation, it said, included sexual intercourse or sexual contact; sexual impropriety comprised "behavior, gestures, or expressions that were seductive, sexually suggestive, or sexually demeaning," such as comments about sexual performance or using the physician-patient relationship to solicit a date. The committee indicated that both types of behavior warranted disciplinary action if a board found that the behavior constituted an "exploitation of the physician-patient relationship."[75]

Sexual contact can occur outside physicians' offices, often in the context of a personal relationship that is concurrent with but independent of treatment.[76] A series of so-called boundary violations usually precedes sexual relations between physicians and patients outside the treatment setting. Physicians start down this "slippery slope" when they change office procedures to spend more time with their "favorite" patients. Examples include scheduling of office appointments for late in the day, lengthy office visits, and numerous telephone calls. Before pursuing a sexual relationship, physicians often exchange gifts with their favorite patients, see them socially, disclose their personal problems to them, and enter into business relationships with them.[77]

Boundary violations often represent the failure of psychiatrists and other mental health professionals to manage properly a phenomenon known as transference. Transference is the unconscious projection by patients of their feelings, desires, and fears from past relationships onto their therapists. When this happens, patients develop strong emotional attachments, leaving them vulnerable to sexual advances. To prevent harming their patients, therapists have to control their own emotional feelings that arise from a parallel phenomenon known as countertransference. Maintaining strict boundary lines is often the best way to offset the effects of countertransference.[78]

Courts have held that physicians who mishandle the transference-countertransference phenomena are guilty of malpractice or gross negligence.[79] Before 1975 there were few lawsuits for sexual misconduct. Since then lawsuits for sexual misconduct have increased substantially, making it a leading cause of malpractice claims against psychotherapists.[80] From about 1984 to 1994, the American Psychiatric Association expelled or suspended 113 of its members for sexual misconduct.[81] In addition, the Federation of State Medical Boards reported that disciplinary actions against physicians for sexual misconduct increased from 84 in 1990 to 132 in 1992.[82]

There are many celebrated cases of physicians who have engaged in sexual relations with patients. For example, Neil Solomon, Maryland's first health secretary and one of its most prominent physicians, surrendered his medical license in 1993 after admitting to sexual "improprieties" with eight female patients over a period of twenty years (*Baltimore Sun*, 31 Oct. 1993). A former deputy medical director of the American Psychiatric Association had his license suspended in 1992 after authorities learned of his two-year relationship with a female patient (*Newsweek*, 13 Apr. 1992). Jules Masserman, past president of the American Psychiatric Association, lost his license to practice medicine in Illinois because a former female patient complained that he "had injected her with barbiturates during treatment and had sex with her while she was unconscious."[83]

Studies show that patients who are victims of sexual misconduct experience guilt, shame, isolation, depression, loss of self-esteem, confusion, fear, and lack of trust.[84] Almost all instances disrupt the therapeutic process.[85] Most patients have difficulty trusting another therapist ever again. Still others attempt suicide and some are successful.[86] Psychologist Kenneth Pope believes that patients who have been sexually abused by their therapists share certain characteristics with those suffering from incest, child abuse, and posttraumatic stress disorder. They may repress their feelings for years, Pope claims, only to encounter them later.[87]

Organized medicine never mounted an aggressive campaign to deal with sexual misconduct as it did with physician substance abuse. There were several reasons for this. First, the profession found it difficult to protect physicians who deliberately violated the physician-patient relationship. Patients under the care of psychiatrists, for instance, often revealed their innermost secrets during therapy. Because of transference, psychiatrists knew that certain patients, particularly those with a history of childhood sexual abuse, were vulnerable to their sexual advances.[88] According to the American Psychiatric Association, sexual exploitation of patients under these circumstances was morally repugnant.[89]

Physicians could reasonably argue that impaired colleagues or poor practitioners did not deliberately exploit their patients for personal gain. Substance abuse was an occupational hazard that adversely affected individual physicians. Substandard care could reflect deficient education and training. The profession claimed that it could address these problems through intervention, rehabilitation, and remediation. The same could not be said for sexual exploitation of vulnerable patients. Law enforcement initiatives were needed to control such activity. Effective self-regulation, though called for, was an inadequate substitute.

Second, there was no clear evidence that treatment programs for physicians who sexually exploited their patients succeeded in altering their behavior.[90] Studies showed that at least one-third of psychiatrists who reported sexual contact with patients were repeat offenders.[91] These physicians were often predators who systematically seduced their patients.[92] Rehabilitation of sexual predators, unlike substance abusers, was not a viable alternative to serious disciplinary action. In such cases, license revocation was the only feasible sanction.[93]

Some cases, however, warranted leniency and retraining. Standards of conduct have evolved considerably in the last twenty years. According to psychologist Gary Schoener, "having a sexual relationship with a former client may, for example, be a more clearly deviant act in 1993 than in 1973."[94] Some older male physicians performed physical examinations that female patients, in particular, considered offensive. Their failure to use chaperons or adequately explain their procedures in advance increased the potential for misunderstanding.[95]

The third reason organized medicine assumed a low profile was the involvement of other occupational groups. Licensing emerged as a public policy issue in the 1970s partly because of the proliferation of the mental health professions.[96] These included psychology, professional and pastoral counseling, social work, and nursing. Since licensure was a precondition to reimbursement under insurance policies, other professionals sought to protect their right to practice under state law.

Infighting among the mental health professions focused attention on psychotherapy and its various dimensions. Since all mental health professionals claimed to be doing "psychotherapy," they also recognized the phenomena of transference and countertransference. When psychologists conducted a study of the incidence of sexual misconduct, their results and conclusions affected psychiatrists, social workers, and other mental health providers. Heightened recognition of the problem across the mental health professions increased media and consumer awareness. Courts determined that therapists who mishandled transference and became sexually involved with their patients committed malpractice. In the case of nonpsychiatric physicians, courts were more lenient.[97] Only the mental health professions were the target of criminal laws in some states.[98]

Finally, the women's movement and the consumer movement altered the terms of the debate. These movements eroded the perception that sexual relations between physicians and their patients were consensual. By focusing on the power imbalance involved, advocates successfully asserted that any sexual activity was exploitative and detrimental. This atmosphere limited the forms of action that professional associations and state medical boards could take. Anything short of expulsion or license revocation might be seen as tolerance of offending physicians.

Despite increasing numbers of disciplinary actions for sexual misconduct since the mid-1980s, consumers were dissatisfied with the level of board activity. Public Citizen complained that "although 67.6% of [doctors surveyed] had actions . . . which took them, at least for awhile, out of the practice of medicine, 32.4%, or almost a third, were allowed to continue practicing, their behavior probably unknown to most of their patients."[99] Complaints like these caused some states to prosecute physicians vigorously for sexual misconduct. Massachusetts was one of those states. As the situation in Massachusetts showed, physicians became politically active when they believed that overzealous enforcement threatened their interests.

The Massachusetts Experience

In 1986 *The Boston Globe* and the television program *60 Minutes* reported that the Massachusetts Board of Registration in Medicine was among the least effective of state medical boards (11 Dec. 1989). Public Citizen ranked the board thirty-ninth out of fifty-one in the number of serious disciplinary actions taken against physicians.[100] The board disciplined a total of seventeen physicians in 1984, twenty-three in 1985, and forty in 1986.[101] According to one of the board's annual reports, its "effectiveness was limited by a professional staff of six, a shoebox filing system and cramped workspace. Hand-processing the license and renewal applications of more than 22,000 physicians was notoriously slow. Out of more than 300 complaints against physicians that were received each year, only the most egregious could be fully investigated and prosecuted by two Board attorneys."[102]

State policy makers viewed the board's ineffectiveness as central to the malpractice insurance crisis that Massachusetts experienced in 1985 and 1986. In 1986 the state expanded the board's budgetary appropriation, allowing it to find new office space, hire attorneys for its disciplinary unit, and computerize its operations.[103] By 1989 the disciplinary unit had fifteen full-time employees, including six investigating attorneys, five prosecuting attorneys, a complaint coordinator, two secretaries, and a unit director.[104]

New resources and personnel meant changed outlooks and expanded capabilities. In just a few short years, the board's ranking improved from thirty-ninth to twentieth (*Boston Globe,* 22 Apr. 1991). Not only could the board review more complaints, it could now handle tougher cases. The board became more vigilant in disciplining physicians guilty of sexually exploiting their patients. Under the leadership of its executive director, Barbara Neuman, the Massachusetts board investigated and prosecuted nineteen psychiatrists for sexual misconduct during 1988 and 1989 (*Boston Globe,* 30 Sept. 1991).

This did not last long. The board's prosecution of high-profile cases involving sexual misconduct alarmed the medical community, creating a backlash. Just as the SCI report inflamed the medical community in New Jersey, so the case of Paul Bettencourt, a specialist in pulmonary disease and internal medicine, served as the "lightning rod" for physician discontent in Massachusetts (*Boston Globe,* 9 Aug. 1990). Relations between the board and the medical community were strained even before the Bettencourt case brought matters to a head. Physicians were particularly distressed about remarks by the chief prosecutor in the board's disciplinary unit at a meeting of the Massachusetts State Bar Association in 1988. According to newspaper accounts, the prosecutor boasted about the powers of the board, proclaiming, "We are the police. We are the prosecution. We are the grand jury and the petit jury. We are the judge and, to a certain extent, even the appellate judge" (*Boston Globe,* 14 Aug. 1990). Although the chair of the board later disavowed these statements, the die was cast. These remarks would serve as a rallying cry for physicians in their struggle with the board over the next several years.

In 1989 the state medical board revoked Bettencourt's license based on allegations that he had sexual relations with a patient (*Boston Globe,* 15 Mar. 1990). Bettencourt denied the allegations and sued the board in federal and state courts. Physicians in Boston's medical community flocked to Bettencourt's side, establishing a defense fund on his behalf. Trustees of the fund mailed out twenty-one thousand copies of a four-page flier detailing the case and warning physicians that "what happened to Dr. Bettencourt could happen to you."[105] Besides supporting Bettencourt financially, physicians petitioned the state legislature to overturn the board's ruling. At a hearing before a legislative committee, several colleagues and patients testified in Bettencourt's favor. The state medical society opposed legislative action, but filed an *amicus* brief with the state's highest court seeking reconsideration of the board's decision (*Boston Globe,* 15 Mar. 1995). As it turned out, special legislation was unnecessary. The appellate court overturned the board's ruling, finding that the record was insufficient to merit revoking Bettencourt's license (*Boston Globe,* 9 Aug. 1990).

Concerted action against the board took its toll. In 1989 the state medical society successfully sponsored legislation that shifted the board's authority to hear disciplinary cases to another state agency (*Boston Globe,* 14 Dec. 1989). It also supported legislation prohibiting the board from disciplining doctors for complaints that were more than six years old. Pressure to curb prosecutions for sexual misconduct led to Barbara Neuman's ouster in 1990 (*Boston Globe,* 3 May 1990). Budget cuts in that same year decimated the board's staff by two-thirds.[106] From 1991 to 1993, the board opened only nine cases against psychiatrists for sexual misconduct (*Boston Globe,* 4 Oct. 1994). During 1990 and most of 1991, it prosecuted one psychiatrist while twelve other cases against psychiatrists remained unresolved. The board's overall ranking again dropped to thirty-ninth (*Boston Globe,* 31 Sept. 1991).

Frustrated with the board's declining level of performance, patients turned to the courts for relief. On the advice of victim's organizations, patients filed more than forty cases against physicians in state courts in Massachusetts in the early 1990s. According to a *Boston Globe* survey conducted in 1994, thirty-eight of these cases resulted in monetary damages averaging $417,000 per claim (4 Oct.). In addition, a broad coalition consisting of victims of sexual misconduct, politicians, and health-care professionals supported legislation in Massachusetts making sexual relations between therapists and patients grounds for criminal prosecution (*Boston Globe,* 24 Jan. 1990). Proponents of criminalization argued that legislative action was necessary to deter sexual misconduct. Opponents asserted that if criminal laws were enacted, reporting would decline even further, and insurers would refuse to pay malpractice claims because most insurance policies excluded coverage for criminal behavior.[107] Although criminalization failed in Massachusetts, it succeeded in a number of other states, including California, Colorado, Connecticut, Florida, Georgia, Iowa, Maine, Minnesota, New Hampshire, New Mexico, North Dakota, South Dakota, Texas, and Wisconsin.[108]

In Massachusetts and elsewhere, recognition of sexual misconduct as a serious problem weakened the resistance of organized medicine to board initiatives. If boards failed to vigorously prosecute physicians for sexual misconduct, consumers served notice that they would seek redress elsewhere. Because of changing attitudes, physicians could no longer ignore the problem. Just as IPPs alleviated concerns about substance abuse, disciplinary action against physicians who sexually exploited their patients was needed to mollify consumers.

Although organized medicine was skeptical about reliance on state boards to curtail sexual misconduct, its options were limited. Since no evidence existed that treatment programs were successful in deterring such behavior, consumers could make a strong case for "zero tolerance."[109] Once organized medicine determined that boards provided a reasonable alternative to the criminal courts, it came to their support. By 1994 even the state medical society in Massachusetts had moved to create a consumer information unit at the state board. The director of government relations for the state medical society called the transformation "revolutionary" (*Boston Globe,* 7 Dec. 1994).

Consumers could now look to boards for protection against wayward physicians. Although organized medicine sometimes resisted, as in Massachusetts, boards showed they could act on their own to manage sexual misconduct cases with little assistance from law enforcement or state medical societies. Still, few accolades came their way. Boards had much to do before consumers accepted them as the profession's "watchdogs." Although they were making some headway, boards still struggled in the 1990s with complaints involving physician incompetence, a problem that neither organized medicine nor federal agencies seemed willing to address. Unless boards stepped into the breach, rapid changes in health-care delivery would eventually limit their authority.

Disciplining Physicians for Professional Incompetence

Like other professionals, physicians claim authority as members of a collegial body to validate their own competence.[110] Those lacking the requisite medical education and training, physicians assert, can neither practice medicine nor assess the competence of those who do.[111] Despite these claims, changes in the medical field over the last thirty years have undermined the exclusive right physicians once had to determine the nature and quality of medical work. Today, nonphysicians often oversee quality assurance programs in hospitals and other health-care facilities. Nonphysicians often decide the level of reimbursement for medical services, and formulate treatment protocols. Nonphysicians also often take an active role in disciplining physicians for incompetence.[112]

The perception that physicians were doing a poor job of policing themselves encouraged federal and state governments to become involved in quality control. Lack of self-discipline, some claimed, was a root cause of the malpractice insurance crisis.[113] Arnold Relman, editor of the *New England Journal of Medicine,* estimated that at least twenty thousand grossly incompetent or negligent doctors were practicing in the United States as of 1984 (*New York Times,* 2 Feb. 1986). Consumer organizations attributed the deaths or injuries of almost two hundred thousand patients each year to poor hospital care.[114]

Pressure on government to do something about rising costs and substandard care led to the formation of professional standards review organizations (PSROs) in 1972 and peer review organizations (PROs) in 1982. On several occasions during the 1970s and 1980s, organized medicine called for their elimination.[115] Although efforts to do so failed, organized medicine profoundly influenced program implementation. Neither PSROs nor PROs were given power to deny payment under the Medicare program for substandard care until 1985.[116] Organized medicine eventually thwarted attempts by federal regulators to identify and eliminate poor practitioners through random case review.[117]

By the early 1990s the federal government had almost stopped disciplining physicians for substandard care. PROs recommended punitive action against a total of twelve physicians in 1991 and fourteen in 1992.[118] Embracing the concept of continuous quality improvement (CQI), PROs became "guide dogs," not "watchdogs." Rather than police the profession, they sought to improve the overall performance of its members through the collection and analysis of data on medical outcomes and practice patterns.[119] Although this educational approach captured the spirit of the quality improvement movement, it failed to alleviate concerns about incompetent practitioners.[120]

A central problem with physician incompetence was determining when and where it existed. Although regulators saw malpractice cases as indicators of poor performance, physicians often complained that reliance on them to assess competence was unfair. They pointed out that insurance companies settled many cases for nuisance value or costs of litigation and that juries decided against physicians because of sympathy for plaintiffs. Many suits were without merit, they said, while others involved errors of judgment or mistakes made under extraordinary circumstances. Moreover, patients sued certain specialists, such as neurosurgeons or obstetricians, more often than others for reasons unrelated to incompetence.[121]

A study conducted under the auspices of Harvard University supported many of these claims. The study indicated that the connection between victim compensation and physician incompetence was tenuous. After reviewing thousands of discharge records from New York hospitals in

1984, researchers concluded that there were few deserving victims of medical negligence and many undeserving ones. Most instances of medical negligence, moreover, involved "slips of the hand or momentary inattention" that were difficult to avoid. Researchers discovered that few cases of medical malpractice involved repeat offenders.[122]

Despite these findings, medical malpractice and physician discipline became closely intertwined. Physicians who wanted tort reform agreed to bolster discipline (*New York Times*, 3 July 1986). Those seeking immunity protection from antitrust lawsuits also agreed that the federal government could collect and maintain information from malpractice insurers, hospitals, and state medical boards in a national data bank.[123] In some states, such as Maryland, three or more malpractice claims triggered an investigation for incompetence.[124]

Confusion over the nature and dimensions of physician incompetence plagued disciplinary bodies. Grad and Marti's study in the late 1970s reported that twenty-seven states used "malpractice" or "gross malpractice" as grounds for disciplinary action while thirty-seven other states employed the terms *medical incompetence, incapacity in the practice of medicine,* or *substandard practice.* Only three states, they discovered, defined the term *incompetence.* Grad and Marti concluded that vague and imprecise standards encouraged inconsistent applications and judicial review.[125]

Boards had to refine their approach. Was "incompetence" the appropriate standard to use for disciplinary purposes, or was it substandard care? How should boards define incompetence and implement their definition? Were multiple acts of negligence required to support a finding of incompetence or were single acts of negligence enough? To what extent were malpractice cases useful indicators of incompetence? Should boards conduct office visits of questionable practitioners and review patient charts at random to determine incompetence? What types of disciplinary action were appropriate and under what circumstances? The answers to these and other questions affected the allocation of limited resources and reliance of boards on outside entities or individuals to collect and analyze information.[126]

Disciplinary actions against physicians for incompetence were so sporadic during the 1970s and 1980s that medical boards were not taken seriously as agents of quality assurance.[127] Identifying and prosecuting physicians for incompetence was time-consuming, expensive, and often controversial.[128] Although boards sought to avoid such cases, they were under constant pressure to do something about them. Government reports were often critical,[129] as were consumer groups and the media.[130] The decision by the federal government to end random case review under the Medicare program placed the burden squarely on the boards. The question was whether boards could meet the challenge. Many were hopeful that they could. The OIG's Mark Yessian believed that boards were the best instrument to hold individual physicians accountable for their negligent conduct.[131] Others agreed, including Sidney Wolfe, executive director of the Public Citizen Health Research Group, and James Winn, executive director of the Federation of State Medical Boards.[132]

Developing the capacity to investigate and prosecute physicians for incompetence required substantial resources, including medical experts to review the information collected and interview practitioners. Unless boards hired their own experts, they had to rely on others to do it for them and report the results. Although peer review was the customary means for evaluating the provision of medical services in hospitals and other health-care facilities, reluctance to use it for disciplinary purposes was widespread. Few physicians relished the adverse consequences that often flowed from criticizing fellow colleagues. Peer reviewers who uncovered instances of poor medical care sometimes encountered hostility, loss of referrals, and lawsuits.[133]

Organized medicine advanced peer review as an educational device, not as a means for disciplinary action. Just as medical societies developed IPPs for purposes of rehabilitation, so they founded peer review programs for purposes of remediation. In calling for the elimination of government-sponsored peer review, the AMA instructed one of its standing committees, the Council on Medical Service, to establish principles for voluntary peer review. Among the principles the council promulgated were the following:

> Medical peer review is a local process.
>
> Physicians are ultimately responsible for all peer review of medical care.
>
> Physicians involved in peer review should be representatives of the medical community. . . .
>
> Peer review of medical practice and the patterns of medical practice of individual physicians . . . is an ongoing process of assessment and evaluation.
>
> Peer review is an educational process for physicians to assure quality medical services.
>
> Any peer review process must protect the confidentiality of medical information obtained and used in conducting peer review.[134]

These principles captured the political underpinnings of professional autonomy. If physicians were to control their own work and the work of others in the medical field, they required full authority to evaluate and assess the quality of medical services in their local communities. Corporations and government agencies threatened to undermine this authority through utilization review and quality assurance programs.[135] Voluntary peer review became the principal vehicle for maintaining the status quo.

The Maryland Experience

Peer review committees of state and local medical societies appeared around the early 1970s. They often succeeded grievance committees that had been struggling to stay afloat under threat of federal antitrust regulation. State and local medical societies had formed grievance committees in the early 1950s to defend physicians against patient complaints. Now they formed peer review committees to defend physicians against the growing intrusion of third parties, including government and insurance carriers.[136] Physicians who established the Peer Review Committee of the Baltimore City Medical Society in 1971 were clear about their intentions. The committee's chairman wrote that the "chief function will be to review, survey, inquire, and recommend the presence of, or changes for optimal physician function. The concern of the committee will be educative rather than censorious. We feel that the province of the committee is to improve the physicians' capability and functioning rather than ferret out the rascals."[137]

Protecting the interests of individual practitioners would be paramount. The Peer Review Committee of the Baltimore City Medical Society would "defend members against unjust allegations" and "establish standards of good practice and countermand any external forces in conflict with those standards." After all, the committee said, peer review was not "a police action" or "a utilization review process for the benefit of third party payors."[138] Maryland's state medical society, known as the Medical and Chirurgical Faculty or simply Med Chi, agreed. In 1974 it adopted the following resolution: "No physician licensed to practice medicine and while practicing medicine in the State of Maryland should be required to reimburse any third party payor all or any portion of fees he has received for services rendered in good faith unless such services have been judged by the physician's peers to be in distinct and proven violation of acceptable standards of medical care."[139]

Because medical societies in Maryland formed peer review committees to protect physicians from the scrutiny of corporate and governmental entities, they were not interested in punishment. Nor were they interested in developing formal standards for peer review.[140] Yet this is precisely what they were supposed to do under Maryland law. Changes to Maryland's Medical Practice Act in 1968 made state and local medical societies agents of the state board. The changes required that the board refer all cases to state and local societies for investigation. Upon completing their investigation, societies were to furnish the board with written reports. Reports were to "contain such recommendations as the investigation reveals might be necessary for adequate disciplinary procedures."[141] How could professional associations in Maryland reconcile their responsibilities under the law with the position that peer review was not intended to "ferret out the rascals"?

Tensions over the proper role of professional associations and the Maryland board in the peer review process divided the medical community. Board members, who were physicians, struggled to balance education and discipline. When the board proposed consolidating peer review at the state level to streamline the process, the president of one local society responded:

> Nowhere in [state law] do I find a legal basis for the [board] becoming a monolithic determiner and interpreter of the inherently vague and constantly changing term "quality medical care," let alone becoming an organization to keep dossiers on every minute detail of every physician's type of practice, hours, size of office, schedules, patient satisfaction or dissatisfaction, ad infinitum. Nor does such a role appear intended for the [board] in carrying out the legal mandate to properly "supervise" and "control" professional conduct (really misconduct). Neither does the creation of any such governmental agency seem necessary or desirable.[142]

Despite resistance from medical societies, government bureaucracy transformed physician peer review as did complex procedural requirements. Physicians under investigation by peer review bodies in Maryland increasingly engaged legal counsel to represent them.[143] Medical societies could do little when attorneys accompanied their clients to "informal" interviews.[144] Right to counsel and other constitutional guarantees were changing the process, and physicians had to keep pace.

By 1980 medical societies in Maryland had developed guidelines for peer reviewers investigating poor practitioners. These guidelines included formal procedures for conducting office visits, interviewing physicians, and obtaining medical records. Reviewers were to recommend possible sanctions and provide sufficient information in their reports to support potential disciplinary action.[145] Few reports, however, recommended sanctions. Because the focus of peer review was education rather than punishment, reviewers failed to weed out incompetent practitioners, as did the state board whose members, all physicians, favored rehabilitation.

By the late 1980s the tension between education and prosecution came to a head. In 1988 a reporter from the *Washington Post,* Susan Schmidt, outlined perceived weaknesses in Maryland's system for disciplining physicians (10, 11 Jan.). She discovered that the state board had revoked the licenses of only eighteen doctors since 1968, two of them for poor patient care. A graphic example was George Richards, a radiologist, who had been sued more than thirty times for negligent treatment of cancer patients. The medical community, Schmidt revealed, had been aware since the late 1960s that Richards's aggressive use of radiation therapy to treat cancer patients had led to instances of serious disfigurement and even death. The state board finally acted in 1980, placing Richards on supervised probation and barring him from treating cancer patients. After a one-year hiatus, the board restored Richards's license in full, though he apparently never again used radiation therapy. Richards's own attorney agreed that the board should have acted sooner to regulate his medical practice (11 Jan.).

Schmidt's articles escalated the controversy that had started a year earlier in Maryland over the close relationship between the state board and organized medicine. A broad coalition of consumers, politicians, and plaintiffs' attorneys sought to end the involvement of Med Chi and local medical societies in peer review. They claimed that other states used nonphysicians to decide cases based on the testimony of medical experts.[146] But in Maryland, as in New Jersey and Massachusetts, organized medicine blunted efforts to overhaul the disciplinary process. Although the state legislature changed the law in 1988 to alter the composition of the board and require greater use of investigators, attorneys, and hearing officers, Med Chi still played a leading role.[147] Under the new law, Med Chi continued to perform peer review in quality-of-care cases. It even enhanced its position vis-à-vis other professional associations. The new law required that all cases targeted by the board for peer review would go directly to Med Chi. Local societies were excluded unless Med Chi decided otherwise.

Even so, Med Chi would pay a price for its continued involvement in physician peer review. For the next several years, consumers, politicians, and the media focused their attention on the state board and the disparate entities now connected with it, including the Office of Attorney General and the Office of Administrative Hearings.[148] In this politically charged atmosphere, maintaining control and avoiding blame were principal considerations. No other system for processing cases in Maryland required the coordination of so many different entities to resolve a single case.[149] Indeed, only Maryland and Connecticut used a private professional association to conduct formal peer review of quality-of-care cases.[150] Because of its unique position, Med Chi was an easy target for criticism. In 1991 state auditors recommended that the legislature abolish the requirement that the board refer quality-of-care cases to Med Chi for peer review.[151] Med Chi either had to focus on discipline or withdraw from the peer review process.

Emphasis on quantity, or numbers of physicians disciplined, now guided the conduct of board members and state officials. Consumer organizations and the media used the rate of discipline in each state to measure board success.[152] Boards that disciplined large numbers of physicians received higher rankings than those that did not. State officials stressed consumer rankings in drafting reports for government agencies or legislative bodies.[153] Although the Federation of State Medical Boards warned that rankings could be misleading, it also listed the number of disciplinary actions for each state in its annual reports released to the media.[154]

Between 1986 and 1994, Maryland's ranking among state medical boards jumped from forty-second to twenty-first.[155] Bernadette Lane, Executive Director of the Baltimore City Medical Society, complained that fixation on numbers was detrimental to both physicians and consumers. The board, she said, now controlled the flow of cases and restricted peer reviewers to examining records and determining whether physicians met standards of care. Direct communication between physicians and peer reviewers rarely occurred. According to Lane, "We're not allowed to tell the physician that we found something wrong in his practice so a year from now or six months from now when the board gets our report the guy is still practicing the same way. I mean if he's doing bad stuff he's still doing bad stuff until the board a year or two from now gets to our report and gets a conference with him. . . . *The difference is that it's now a legal procedure when it used to be a procedure of education*" (italics added).[156]

Before the 1980s, peer review focused on the hospital setting. Now government, consumers, and insurance carriers used peer review to control the cost and quality of medical services in any setting, including physicians' private offices. Rather than review the work of their colleagues to satisfy professional concerns, physicians did it to satisfy the concerns of others. Peer review became more formal, more centralized, more public, and more punitive. Peer reviewers answered to nonphysician administrators of hospitals, insurance companies, managed-care organizations, and disciplinary bodies. The attitudes of physicians also changed. Quality assurance still stressed education, but physicians recognized that cost control and discipline were essential components of peer review. Physicians who long balked at efforts to "ferret out the rascals" now took part in these endeavors.

Conclusion

Schattschneider viewed politics in the United States as a struggle between two competing power systems, business and government. He observed that dominant interests seek private settlements because they can control the outcome, whereas weaker interests appeal to public authority for redress of private grievances.[157] The three case studies included in this chapter support Schattschneider's thesis.

In the case of physicians who abused drugs and alcohol, organized medicine promoted IPPs as a viable alternative to disciplinary action. When these programs failed to appraise state medical boards of dangerous practitioners, as in New Jersey, an investigative body charged that physicians had engaged in a "conspiracy of silence." In the case of physicians who sexually exploited their patients, media and consumer interests pressed boards to discipline offenders. When the state medical board in Massachusetts increased prosecutions, organized medicine lobbied the state legislature to curb the board's powers. In the case of physicians who were incompetent or practiced below the standard of care, organized medicine advanced peer review as an educational device. When peer review became central to the investigation of practitioners for substandard care, as in Maryland, consumer groups and the press raised a conflict of interest.

Victims of physician impairment, sexual misconduct, and incompetence turned to the press, the courts, state legislatures, and state agencies for redress of their complaints. Organized medicine responded in the 1970s and 1980s with IPPs and peer review committees, just as it had in the 1950s with grievance committees of state and local medical societies. IPPs and peer review committees channeled conflict in directions more palatable to physicians: remediation and rehabilitation rather than formal discipline and public disclosure. If private remedies failed, physicians sometimes used political muscle to stem zealous enforcement.

State medical boards evolved during the 1970s and 1980s through efforts to reconcile public and professional concerns. They tempered bureaucracy with professionalism, discipline with rehabilitation, and disclosure with confidentiality. Although not the most efficient mechanisms for managing large caseloads, boards served the interests of key actors in the medical field. By the time the turbulent 1980s were over, most boards and professional associations had resolved their differences and enhanced their oversight of the medical profession. Just as they seemed to be getting their act together, however, managed care introduced a new set of problems and concerns.

CHAPTER FIVE

The Battle with HMOs

Market competition in health care challenged the viability of regulatory agencies such as state medical boards just as it did that of organized medicine and related institutions. Efforts to control the costs of medical services shifted political power from providers to payers of health care with remarkable speed. Insurance companies and large corporate employers reorganized the medical field to reflect their interests as risk-takers and third-party payers. They asserted that an integrated delivery system, composed of networks of physicians and hospitals, could reduce costs while sustaining or even improving overall quality. Large, for-profit companies came to dominate the health-care industry; physicians no longer exercised monopoly powers. Although physicians often held influential positions within managed-care organizations, they relinquished control over medical decision making to the organizations themselves.[1]

Corporate administrators of HMOs used several devices to lower costs and increase profits. They replaced fee-for-service with capitation as the principal method of compensating physicians. Because most physicians received a fixed sum for each patient, they had little incentive to overspend. Administrators also introduced utilization review to evaluate treatment plans. Reviewers could deny coverage for care they deemed medically unnecessary or inappropriate. Finally, administrators used primary-care physicians as gatekeepers to limit access to specialists and other medical services.

These various cost-cutting devices placed physicians in an awkward position. For some, their role as patient advocate collided with their role as corporate employee. Although traditional institutions and supporting legal doctrine stressed professional autonomy, the tide favored corporate accountability. Institutions and laws that bolstered professional control had been under attack since the federal government had fostered managed care in the early 1970s. State medical boards were among several targets.

Managed-care organizations threatened state medical boards in several ways. Foremost was the notion that federal and state lawmakers should eliminate or revise laws protecting physicians' "scope of practice." Cost-cutting advocates opposed laws that restricted the use of alternative providers who, they claimed, increased access to and decreased costs of medical services.[2] Eliminating or modifying such laws would undercut the authority of state medical boards to police medicine's boundaries. Another threat concerned the reduced autonomy of physicians in medical decision making. Utilization review practices of managed-care organizations added another layer to the decision-making process. Boards now had to determine whether and how to apply the grounds for medical discipline to physician managers of corporate providers that denied coverage for medical services. Managed-care organizations also challenged the criteria for judging the performance of physicians by shifting the focus from individual to population-based care.[3] Efforts of HMOs to ration medical services were in conflict with professional standards and values. Finally, the process for certifying physicians to managed-care panels heightened resistance to medical discipline. Because managed-care panels often excluded physicians based on disciplinary action, boards discovered that formal discipline, even of a remedial nature, jeopardized a physician's career.

Organized medicine, potential losers, appealed to consumer groups and the press to support legislation that curtailed the corporate practice of medicine. As part of the ever-widening conflict, state medical boards pursued means for bringing managed care under their purview. By regulating utilization review activities of HMOs, boards expanded their jurisdiction into areas that corporate medicine now controlled.

The Threat to State Licensure Laws

Federal policy favored reorganization of medical services under the banner of managed care, and federal agencies promoted the concept in several ways. For example, the Agency for Health Care Policy and Research developed guidelines or protocols to standardize the practice of medicine.[4] The National Practitioner Data Bank collected background information on physicians to streamline the credentialing process.[5] The Federal Trade Commission invoked antitrust laws to thwart concerted attempts by independent practitioners to compete with managed-care organizations.[6]

When President Clinton sought to reform the health-care system in 1993, he attempted to build on these prior initiatives. The president's Health Security Act called on federal agencies to formulate practice guidelines and to provide consumers with quality report cards containing comparative information on health-care providers.[7] Organized medicine was apprehensive about these proposals.[8] Practice guidelines reflected the efforts of government researchers to reduce clinical uncertainty. Whereas organized medicine saw them as tools for assisting physicians in diagnosis and treatment, HMOs used them as the basis for third-party reimbursement.[9] Quality report cards or practice profiles measured the performance of individual practitioners and institutional providers. Organized medicine championed their educational value; HMOs used them to weed out doctors who failed to satisfy their criteria for economy and efficiency.[10]

President Clinton's plan also attempted to dismantle the federal peer review program and to override state licensing laws.[11] Section 1161 of the proposed Health Security Act stated that "no State may, through licensure or otherwise, restrict the practice of any class of health professionals beyond what is justified by the skills and training of such professionals."[12] Commentators suggested that this provision constituted "a fundamental assault on the physicians' citadel."[13] In one bold stroke, President Clinton sought to alter traditional means of regulating practitioners of medicine by eliminating professional barriers to task performance.

The Federation of State Medical Boards was alarmed. In testimony before Congress, the federation's executive vice president, James Winn, claimed that if section 1161 were enacted into law, it would "likely cause a complete upheaval of the health provider regulatory scheme." Winn asserted that state licensure laws provided the most reliable framework for judging competence. The proposed act, he said, created confusion about the validity of those laws. He predicted that the provision would encourage lawsuits against state boards from those seeking to overturn traditional restrictions on scope of practice.[14]

Actually President Clinton's proposal contained nothing new. According to a report prepared by the federal government in 1971, occupational licensure prevented hospitals and other health-care facilities from making optimal use of their personnel. These institutions, the report maintained, required more flexibility in responding to rapid change in the medical field. By eliminating barriers to task performance, health-care facilities could assign jobs based on skill, education, and in-service training.[15]

Debate over the Health Security Act resurrected the concept of institutional licensure and other mechanisms for regulating the practice of medicine in large-scale organizations.[16] Although Congress failed to enact the Health Security Act, the issue concerning state scope-of-practice laws did not go away. In 1995 a task force of the Pew Health Professions Commission also recommended that restrictions on scope of practice be abolished. Although the task force did not propose an end to individual licensure and discipline, it recommended that states consider increasing the level of public and interdisciplinary representation on state boards. It also suggested that states examine techniques for coordinating efforts among professional boards to reflect the current emphasis on "'continuum of care' rather than discrete services provided by individual professionals."[17]

Even if scope-of-practice laws remained unchanged, the die was cast. More flexible boundaries accommodated an emerging system that stressed primary care, not specialty care; ambulatory care, not institutional care; and preventive care, not costly treatments and interventions. Just as managed care required fewer physicians to support these cost-saving and gatekeeping techniques, so it relied on nonphysicians, such as nurse practitioners, nurse midwives, and physician assistants to provide medical services. Teams consisting of primary-care physicians and their nonphysician extenders furnished the multiple skills required to manage a patient population in an efficient and effective manner.[18] By virtue of its dominant position in certain markets, managed care influenced the work rules for various health-care professions, and boards adjusted to these new realities.[19]

Several other issues remained on the table in the wake of the failed Clinton plan: formulation of practice guidelines, collection and dissemination of information on providers, and oversight of quality in integrated systems. The plan proposed that the federal government coordinate these efforts under the auspices of a National Health Board.[20] Upon the failure of the Clinton plan, state agencies, organized medicine, and managed-care organizations tangled over these issues.

Cost versus Quality

By the early 1990s managed-care organizations dominated the health-care markets in several regions of the United States, particularly along the East and West Coasts.[21] Large HMOs, such as U.S. Healthcare and Wellpoint Health Networks, became even larger by merging with traditional insurers like Massachusetts Mutual. Although these so-called megadeals were reminiscent of corporate takeovers during the 1980s, they were friendly acquisitions that favored the smaller HMOs.[22] Monopoly and oligopoly characterized the situation in major population centers.

Taking advantage of their superior bargaining position in certain markets, HMOs gained control over physician selection and retention, methods of compensation, and even the nature and content of communications between physicians and their patients.[23] For boards, the methods that HMOs used to "deselect" physicians from their panels was particularly vexing. Boards had struggled for many years to improve their level of performance while balancing professional and public concerns. In several instances, this meant taking formal action that was remedial in nature. HMOs threatened this delicate balance by excluding physicians from their panels for even minor transgressions.[24] Keenly aware of the possible consequences, some boards declined formal action or reverted to private solutions.[25]

Under siege, the profession's leaders went on the offensive. Cost-conscious corporations, they asserted, could not be trusted to protect the interests of plan participants. Physicians were needed to ensure that patients received optimal care. Leonard Laster, a professor of medicine and health policy at the University of Massachusetts Medical Center, proclaimed that "to restore quality we must set strict limits on how far health care managers are allowed to go in reaching for profits. Patients should join with groups of doctors, nurses and consumers to pull the health care pendulum back toward the patient's interests. We must define the conditions for managed care, and we must impose restrictions and accountability on the players."[26]

Organized medicine, assuming the initiative, seized every opportunity to emphasize the threat to quality from for-profit corporations. Several practices of managed-care organizations were targets of negative publicity. These included premature hospital discharges, restrictions on diagnostic tests and specialty referrals, preauthorization requirements for emergency room care, limitations on treatment for mental illness, and gag clauses in managed-care contracts.[27] The gag clauses often prevented doctors from revealing certain information to their patients about treatment options, facilities, and specialists excluded from managed-care plans.[28]

Consumer groups, welcoming these attacks, joined organized medicine in sponsoring legislation that required HMOs to provide certain benefits, such as longer hospital stays and coverage for emergency services, as well as choices among health plans and providers. They also participated in efforts to temper contractual relations between physicians and managed-care entities, such as laws banning gag clauses and promoting due process protections for physicians fearful of termination.[29]

Many of these attempts were successful.[30] Using the AMA's model Patient Protection Act as a guide, several states enacted legislation that required insurance carriers to provide maternity benefits for minimum hospital stays following delivery.[31] Other states passed any-willing-provider laws that prevented HMOs from excluding doctors from their networks for reasons unrelated to quality of care.[32] State officials in New Jersey proposed rules prohibiting HMOs from interfering in treatment decisions on the basis of cost.[33] State medical societies in New York and elsewhere sought to ban gag clauses.[34] Bad publicity encouraged industry giants, such as U.S. Healthcare, to back down on their own.[35]

Physicians pressed their agenda in other forums as well, including federal and state courts. In New York, anesthesiologists at three hospitals on Long Island, claiming violations of federal antitrust laws, sued Aetna Life and Casualty.[36] In New Hampshire a physician claiming that his termination violated public policy sued an HMO.[37] In Illinois a surgeon resurrected the legal doctrine prohibiting the corporate practice of medicine to defeat a claim filed against him for breach of contract.[38] State medical societies played supporting roles in many of these lawsuits. Adopting a quality-first strategy, physician litigants stressed the adverse effect on patient care if corporate medicine prevailed.

Finally, professional associations sought to preempt efforts by government agencies and HMOs to formulate practice guidelines and to develop indicators of clinical performance. Several associations established practice guidelines that stressed quality over cost.[39] The AMA initiated its own Physician Performance Assessment Program to reduce the emphasis on economics in the credentialing process.[40] Writing in the *New England Journal of Medicine,* Jerome Kassirer observed that "from a system that until recently was dominated by reliance on intelligent and thoughtful decision making by individual doctors, we seem to have embarked on a path of codifying the practice of medicine. In part, we are doing so in the name of quality."[41]

A Matter of Ethics

Organized medicine reasserted itself by successfully portraying physicians as the remaining bridgehead against profit-hungry CEOs and cost-cutting bureaucrats. Consumers found arguments that managed-care organizations, if left unchecked, would eventually undermine the sanctity of physician-patient relationships to be persuasive.[42] Physicians were needed to restore the balance between cost and quality in the provision of medical services. The AMA's Council on Ethical and Judicial Affairs put it bluntly: "No other party in the health care system is charged with the responsibility of advocating for patients, and no other party can reasonably be expected to assume the responsibility conscientiously."[43]

Just as the medical profession fashioned codes of ethics and disciplinary rules to forge a professional order, so it used them to reclaim political power under the new regime. According to the council, managed care posed two main problems for physicians—first, the allocation of scarce resources among patients and second, the creation of financial incentives for physicians to limit patient care.[44] To retain their professional standing, physicians had to resolve these conflicts in ways that benefited their patients.

Before the appearance of managed care, physicians had few incentives to conserve resources beyond ethical prohibitions on wasteful spending and unnecessary treatment. Third-party reimbursement and fear of lawsuits for malpractice reinforced the incentives to exhaust treatment options. Managed care altered this perspective by limiting access to medical services and by reversing financial incentives to overspend. The needs of society were in tension with the needs of individuals under managed care.

Conflicting values created a serious dilemma for physicians. Could doctors ration services to patients yet satisfy their responsibilities as professionals? The council said no. Although it acknowledged that doctors had a duty to protect society's resources, the council asserted that "physicians must remain primarily dedicated to the health care needs of their individual patients." Because medical ethics extolled the welfare of patients, the council warned doctors against withholding treatment in order to preserve the resources of managed-care organizations.[45]

Legal doctrine supported the council's position. Courts held that physicians had a fiduciary duty to their patients to render the best care available under the circumstances. Even proponents of cost control recognized that physicians could not escape their fiduciary obligations unless courts adjusted the standard of care to accommodate the economic interests of society. Some legal scholars argued that courts should do just that. They noted that standards of care were flexible, that they responded to changes in medical custom and practice. Recent abandonment of the locality rule in most jurisdictions was an example. Courts, they said, should take into consideration the likely adverse effects of increased tort liability on cost-containment policies.[46]

Despite frequent attempts to reform the tort liability system, organized medicine opposed alteration of the standard of care. Since the standard of care protected the interests of individual patients at the expense of society, physicians believed that it counterbalanced cost-containment measures of managed-care organizations. According to the AMA's Board of Trustees, changing the legal standard might lead to rationing and degradation of quality.[47]

Organized medicine sought not only to preserve the standard of care but also to apply it to utilization review decisions of third-party payers. Imposing legal liability was a means of holding managed-care organizations accountable for the adverse consequences of cost-containment policies. After all, courts expected doctors to meet the standard of care even if HMOs failed to authorize payment.[48] As Leonard Laster observed, "a dose of legal liability could be a very effective way to draw the attention of the insurance administrators to issues of quality."[49]

The *Darling* case, decided in 1965, imposed liability on hospitals for the conduct of medical staff.[50] Now it was imposed on managed care. Few state courts had difficulty extending the concept of vicarious liability to HMOs. Whether patients could sue HMOs for medical malpractice when they denied coverage for medical services was another matter.[51] The answer often depended on the type of health-care plan involved.

Beginning with the 1986 case of *Wickline v. State of California*,[52] state courts in California took managed care to task. The plaintiff in *Wickline* claimed that her premature discharge from the hospital following surgery led to serious complications and eventual amputation of her right leg. Although the court in *Wickline* found that there had been no breach of the standard of care, it proclaimed that "third party payers of health care services can be held legally accountable when medically inappropriate decisions result from defects in the design or implementation of cost containment mechanisms."[53]

In *Wilson v. Blue Cross of Southern California*, the California court followed through on its earlier reasoning, holding that a wrongful death action against Blue Cross for refusing to extend treatment for depression and drug dependency could proceed to trial.[54] Finally, in *Fox v. Health Net*, a California jury in 1993 awarded $12 million in compensatory damages and $77 million in punitive damages against an HMO for failing to authorize a bone marrow transplant for a patient with advanced breast cancer.[55] State courts in other jurisdictions also inched toward extending legal liability to HMOs for medical injuries caused by their cost-containment policies.[56]

Blocking their way, however, was the federal Employer Retirement Income Security Act of 1974 (ERISA).[57] ERISA preempted state regulations concerning employee-benefit plans, including health plans of self-insured employers. Although many disputed Congress's intent to interfere with state and local laws directed against poor treatment decisions, managed-care organizations claimed otherwise, asserting the need for uniformity.[58] Because nearly two-thirds of employer health plans qualified for ERISA preemption, ERISA provided managed-care organizations with a potent weapon in their struggle against state and local regulation. Federal courts even invoked ERISA to strike down state laws modeled on portions of the AMA's Patient Protection Act.[59]

Because ERISA precluded recovery for compensatory and punitive damages, HMOs removed cases to federal courts when sued for medical malpractice. They claimed that utilization review was an administrative activity that related to the operation of an employee-benefit plan. Accordingly, HMOs argued that ERISA preempted any state lawsuit seeking damages for the adverse consequences of cost-containment decisions. Although federal courts initially split on this issue, the weight of authority favored HMOs.[60] In *Corcoran v. United Healthcare, Inc.*,[61] for example, the U.S.

Court of Appeals for the Fifth Circuit held that ERISA preempted plaintiff's wrongful death action for denial of medical services following a high-risk pregnancy. The court expressed dissatisfaction with its own decision, observing that the result eliminated an important check on managed-care organizations.

By the mid-1990s public backlash against managed care began to sway court doctrine. Two Supreme Court rulings, the first in 1995 and the second in 1997, afforded states the right to regulate medical services of self-insured plans. Subsequent opinions of lower federal courts now conceded that ERISA did not bar lawsuits against HMOs when they denied coverage for medical services.[62] Texas became the first state in 1997 to pass legislation giving plan participants the right to sue HMOs for medical malpractice. Aetna Health Plans of Texas filed suit to block the initiative, arguing that health costs would increase unless ERISA preempted such legislation. Physicians responded, claiming that a distinction existed between medical and administrative decision making, and that utilization review encompassed the former, not the latter. Some members of Congress agreed with physicians and sought to amend ERISA to exclude lawsuits for medical malpractice.[63] State medical boards carefully monitored these events, as they dueled HMOs over regulation of utilization review activities.

Penetrating the "Corporate Veil" of Managed Care

Like other components of the professional order, state medical boards operated under the assumption that physicians were in charge. This simplified the disciplinary process. When patients received poor care, boards did not have to look very far. The major consideration was the quality of care that treating physicians provided.

Managed care altered this assumption. Because many doctors now functioned within a corporate hierarchy, holding them responsible for poor patient care was problematic. Medical decision making was part of a bureaucratic process that involved nonphysician providers and administrative personnel. As a result, state medical boards struggled to determine professional accountability. Proposals to override state scope-of-practice laws and to abolish government-sponsored peer review were logical extensions of an integrated delivery system. State medical boards sought to survive in this new climate by penetrating the "corporate veil" of managed care and by joining forces with organized medicine to protect the public interest.

Until recently, state medical boards had encountered little resistance from third-party payers in their efforts to regulate the practice of medicine. Although state statutes defined "practice of medicine" broadly to include almost anything related to patient care, boards did not pursue physicians who engaged in utilization review before the 1990s. Utilization review was something that hospitals and insurance companies did to evaluate the necessity and appropriateness of patient care. The process took on new meaning when managed-care organizations used it to withhold treatment. Now that courts had begun to impose legal liability for cost containment, boards sought to impose similar duties on licensees.

In several states, including Arizona, Maryland, and Minnesota, boards first attempted to obtain legislative approval for disciplinary action against physician reviewers.[64] HMOs vigorously opposed these efforts, arguing that utilization review was an administrative function that other government agencies already addressed.[65] The medical director of one HMO did not mince words. He viewed proposed legislation in Maryland as "pure and simple an attack on managed care."[66] Because the statutory agent in Maryland for determining "appropriate standards" was the state medical society, he was not far off the mark. Had the legislation passed, the state medical society would have gained authority to review adverse medical decisions of Maryland HMOs.

Lack of similar legislation in Arizona did not deter the state medical board. In 1994 it reproached the medical director of Blue Cross/Blue Shield, John Murphy, for failing to authorize gallbladder surgery for a patient. The patient's surgeon had complained to the board that Murphy's actions constituted "unprofessional conduct and/or medical incompetence."[67] Murphy responded to the complaint by saying that "as Medical Director of Blue Cross and Blue Shield of Arizona, I am not involved in patient care and not involved in the practice of medicine. Therefore, I question whether the performance of my duties is subject to the review of the Board of Medical Examiners."[68]

After an investigation, the board voted to issue a "letter of concern" on the grounds that Murphy's actions were "inappropriate" and "could have caused harm to a patient."[69] Before the final version of the letter was in the mail, however, Blue Cross/Blue Shield sued the board on Murphy's behalf, claiming that it lacked authority to investigate "claims handling decisions" of insurance companies.[70] According to Blue Cross/Blue Shield, utilization review was a "business function," not the practice of medicine. The HMO argued that if an investigation was called for, the state insurance commissioner should have exclusive jurisdiction.[71]

The assertion that state insurance departments offered protection from poor decisions of licensed reviewers was a diversion. State insurance departments had power to investigate coverage decisions but lacked medical expertise. Medical boards were the only state government agencies capable of investigating complex medical decisions. Like many other court decisions, this one had major political implications beyond the narrow legal issues involved.

The Arizona trial court held in favor of the board on the jurisdictional issue, and Blue Cross/Blue Shield appealed. The case then received national attention, and major players affected by the controversy chose sides. Representatives of the insurance industry criticized boards for trying to assume yet more responsibilities than they could handle. They also asserted that a conflict of interest existed because physicians stood to gain financially from peer review of coverage decisions.[72] For its part, the Federation of State Medical Boards filed an *amicus* brief with the court. It noted that boards were often patients' only effective remedy when HMOs withheld medical care.[73]

Medical boards across the nation awaited the outcome of the *Murphy* case. They were not disappointed when an appellate court ruled in 1997 that the Arizona board had the authority to review Murphy's actions. According to the court, Murphy's preauthorization denial of coverage for gallbladder surgery was a medical decision, not an insurance decision. The court's ruling confirmed the belief of many physicians that standards affecting practitioners also should apply to insurance companies that engaged in utilization review.[74] Because of the implications of the court's holding, Blue Cross/Blue Shield vowed to appeal.[75]

Boards in other states moved quickly as the controversy played out in Arizona. In four states, boards required medical directors of HMOs to have an in-state medical license.[76] After the ruling in *Murphy,* these boards did not want HMOs to escape their jurisdiction by hiring physicians with out-of-state licenses to perform utilization review. In Florida the state board pursued criminal penalties against the unlicensed medical director of an HMO who engaged in utilization review activities.[77] In Massachusetts the state board attempted to expand reporting requirements for HMOs and related health-care facilities. A state advisory panel even urged that the Massachusetts board be permitted to audit peer review records of health-care facilities to assess the accuracy of reportable information.[78]

These and other efforts were a prelude to future battles. Mark Speicher, executive director of the Arizona board, remarked at the federation's annual convention in 1996 that managed care had thrust boards into a new role, "that of protecting the public from the new dangers imposed by a data- and dollar-driven health-care system."[79] Boards needed allies if they were to take on the managed-care industry, as did organized medicine. State boards and organized medicine seemed willing to put aside past differences for their mutual benefit.

Circling the Wagons

Changes in the medical field drove a wedge between state medical boards and state medical societies in the 1970s. Left to their own devices, many boards obtained the resources and developed the organization to strike out on their own. By the late 1980s the level of disciplinary actions against licensed physicians had increased substantially. Responding to pressure from boards and other government agencies to put its house in order, organized medicine took serious steps toward genuine self-regulation. IPPs were a prime example.

A common enemy now threatened state medical boards and professional associations alike: managed care. Its underlying premise forecast an end to professional autonomy and institutions that supported it. Enticed by the prospects for cost savings, state and federal officials seized on managed care as a panacea for a beleaguered health-care system. In so doing, they overlooked its many blemishes.

Striving to maintain political power and economic clout, leaders of organized medicine sought to recast the professional order. Their rallying cry was "quality." Cost containment, they preached, lowered quality unless government joined with them in refashioning means for professional control. The prescriptions were not much different than before—a self-governing medical staff for managed-care organizations, a national accreditation body controlled by physicians, and mechanisms for safeguarding the traditional doctor-patient relationship.[80]

Medical boards struggled to meet the latter requirement. As Arnold Relman succinctly stated before the Federation of State Medical Boards in 1995:

> The social function of the medical profession is to act as the patient's fiduciary. That's why doctors are licensed. That's why doctors have a license monopoly. That's why their education is subsidized. That's why they have all the benefits and all the advantages and all the protection from competition that society and states afford them when they license them. And in exchange for that license monopoly and that protection from competition and those subsidies, doctors are expected to act as fiduciaries for their patients, to represent the patient's interest.[81]

Following years of inadequate self-regulation, organized medicine sought to regain consumer confidence. Joining forces with state medical boards was one way to show consumers that doctors were serious about quality. Several initiatives demonstrated the profession's desire to court consumers. These efforts ranged from the provision of experts to assist in case investigation to the reinstitution of case mediation.

Maryland supplied the model for cooperative ventures between state medical boards and state medical societies in the investigation of quality-of-care cases. Few states, if any, required boards to collaborate with professional associations in peer review. In 1991 the AMA proposed that other state medical societies assist boards in case investigation.[82] Implementing the proposal was a problem, however, because boards were reluctant to work closely with state medical societies.[83] Years of wrangling over issues such as impaired physicians programs and sexual misconduct cases had discouraged board members and board administrators alike.

In spite of their past differences, fear of managed care drove medical boards and medical societies closer together. The Federation of State Medical Boards in 1994 approved the AMA's proposal with the understanding that boards would have sole responsibility for quality-of-care issues. State medical boards would be a "key element" in the peer review system, responsible for "the most serious quality of care complaints."[84] For the first time, organized medicine sanctioned a punitive role for government-sponsored peer review.

Another important development was progress on case mediation. Many years before, state and local medical society grievance committees had been active in resolving patient complaints. Federal antitrust activity during the 1970s had squelched efforts to mediate complaints involving excessive fees, unprofessional conduct, and substandard care. Noting widespread dissatisfaction on the part of patients with the health-care delivery system, the AMA took steps to revive grievance committees. The AMA revised its guidelines for processing of consumer complaints and petitioned the FTC in 1992 for an advisory opinion on mediation of fee disputes.[85] While limiting the initiative in certain respects, the FTC gave the AMA the green light in 1994 to discipline doctors who engaged in "fee gouging."[86]

The Massachusetts medical board, seeking a way to reduce its growing caseload, also turned to case mediation in 1994. Mediation had several advantages over traditional adjudication. It circumvented the disciplinary process, which was often quite lengthy, and allowed consumers to negotiate a settlement. Many expressed concern, however, that boards might pursue cases that did not merit disciplinary action or might overlook doctors guilty of serious misconduct.[87] Although skeptical, consumer groups generally favored the Massachusetts approach. The Citizen Advocacy Center even touted case mediation for use in other states, including California, Florida, Minnesota, Ohio, and Texas.[88]

Finally, state medical boards and state medical societies began to loosen restrictions on public access to background information on physicians. Recommendations for health-care reform, including those of President Clinton and the Pew Health Professions Commission, often stressed consumer empowerment.[89] Reformers claimed that consumers could protect themselves if they knew more about their doctors. Heretofore, organized medicine had always opposed disclosure of disciplinary data on grounds that consumers might misinterpret the information presented.[90]

Now that managed-care organizations threatened to bury information on insurance coverage by "gagging" doctors, organized medicine softened its opposition to consumer empowerment. State medical boards, which had begun disclosing some disciplinary records, expanded the nature and type of information available to the public.[91] In 1997 the Massachusetts board became the first to disclose certain derogatory information about physicians, including criminal convictions, malpractice payouts, and restrictions on hospital privileges.[92] Even the Massachusetts Medical Society announced its support for the release of information on medical malpractice claims and settlements. Upon learning of the medical society's position, the executive director of the Massachusetts board remarked, "That's a real sea change in their attitude."[93]

It certainly was. Although the Massachusetts Medical Society would eventually seek to refine the information disclosed to consumers, the lesson was clear: health-care policy and politics had abruptly changed in just a few short years. Leaders of organized medicine had perceived the need to alter prior strategies. The signs were evident: genuine self-regulation, consumer-oriented legislation, and cooperative arrangements between state medical boards and state medical societies.

CHAPTER SIX

State Medical Boards
and the New Corporate Order

Alexis de Toqueville once observed that a key feature of American government was the decentralized character of administration. "Written laws exist in America," he wrote, "and one sees the daily execution of them; but although everything moves regularly, the mover can nowhere be discovered. The hand which directs the social machine is invisible."[1] Toqueville could easily have been describing the state of affairs in the health-care industry before the advent of government regulation and corporate reorganization during the 1970s and 1980s.

Under the old regime, physicians were virtually immune from outside scrutiny. Doctors policed their own by means of local institutions they controlled. The hand that regulated the health-care industry, as well as the quality and provision of medical services, was invisible. Under the new regime, physicians were accountable to employers or third-party payers of medical services, such as HMOs or government agencies. External scrutiny became the norm, rather than the exception. Dependent on the professional monopoly for support, the framework for self-regulation eroded, giving way to government and corporate oversight. Inexorably, the visible hand of corporate management replaced the invisible hand of professional self-regulation.[2]

The emergence of modern state medical boards in the 1980s was but one of a series of events that reflected the decline of the former self-governing professional order. Government subsidization of health care through enactment of the Medicare and Medicaid programs in the 1960s enhanced access to medical services and attracted commercial investors who reaped profits from health-care facilities and new technology. During the 1970s and 1980s costs of health care increased as well as complaints for medical malpractice. The former strained the ability of government and employers to balance budgets and satisfy expenses; the latter led to crises in the availability and affordability of medical malpractice insurance. While efforts to contain costs through prospective payment, utilization review, and market competition altered traditional means of financing and delivering medical services, efforts to curb lawsuits for malpractice focused attention on the lack of medical discipline.

Public pressures to contain costs and improve quality politicized the disciplinary process. Application of federal antitrust to the medical field undercut private means of enforcing professional norms and values and of adjusting complaints that patients filed against their physicians. Grievance committees of state and local medical societies and peer review committees of community hospitals operated at their peril in the absence of "state action immunity" or statutory protection. The medical profession's model for resolving complaints, which emphasized collegiality, informality, and confidentiality, became impractical for expediting cases, satisfying requirements of due process, and disclosing information on physician performance.

State governments, courts, consumers, and the press further widened the scope of conflict over medical discipline. Responding to crises in medical malpractice, states placed consumers on board panels, curtailed the authority of medical societies to select physician members, and gained oversight of board operations through budgetary practices and reporting procedures. As in other sectors of the economy, consumers organized to protect their interests and pressed boards to resolve complaints for incompetence and professional misconduct. In the event that boards ignored their concerns, courts, the media, and law enforcement agencies offered alternative means of achieving satisfaction.

But boards would not respond overnight. Organized medicine resisted external oversight, as physicians did any threat to their professional autonomy. State governments had neither the resources nor the scientific basis to mount an attack; the best they could do was impose medical discipline through layers of bureaucracy.

For boards to advance, physicians had to reconcile their interests with those of a pluralist society. The unrelenting demands of new stakeholders challenged traditional mechanisms for resolving disputes. Drastic improvements in case management were needed to satisfy the public's interest in efficiency and neutrality. Physicians in the 1980s were more willing to change board practices and procedures. Unlike their colleagues from earlier generations, they regularly assimilated practices from the business community, including the formalization of professional controls. Unlike their colleagues from earlier generations, they did not resist centralized management and reporting so long as resources and funds flowed in their direction.

The modern state medical board that emerged in the late 1980s and early 1990s reflected the long-standing struggle among contending forces seeking to privatize and socialize conflict. Physicians comprised a majority of each board but delegated much of their authority over routine matters to an operating core consisting of investigators, administrators, and case managers. Lawyers, medical consultants, and hearing officers rounded out the picture, giving boards the ability to resolve difficult and complex cases through settlement agreements or adjudication. Physicians remained in charge, but they shared authority with government bureaucrats, and their principal theater of operation was in the public, not the private, sector.

Since the 1970s, state medical boards had narrowed the gap between the profession they protected and the public they served. But few outside the medical community and the consumer organizations that monitored their performance proclaimed their social worth. The conquering heroes of corporate medicine and the prognosticators of medicine's future viewed boards as irrelevant, at best, or as obstacles to a fully integrated health-care system, at worst.

The Economic Model and Professional Accountability

According to health analyst Mark Peterson, 1994 was a watershed year for the nation's health-care industry.[3] A political cartoon appearing in the *New York Times* on Sunday, November 26, 1996, crystallized the situation: two years after the defeat of the Clinton plan, most consumers, including the fictional characters Harry and Louise who had been featured in television ads against the plan, were in an HMO. The accompanying editorial indicated that where politicians failed, private industry succeeded in cutting costs by closing hospitals and by restricting consumers' right to choose their physician. The failure of the Clinton plan did not reflect support for the old status quo. Rather, Peterson claimed that federal inaction "unleashed a private sector initiative that literally transformed the status of patients, the physician-patient relationship, interactions among different types of providers, the meaning and role of insurance, and the very structure of health delivery and financing institutions."[4] What did the success of corporate medicine mean for state medical boards? Who would police managed-care organizations?

Corporate integration of the health-care industry created multiple levels of accountability, from managed-care plans to institutional providers to individual physicians.[5] Traditional means used to regulate physician behavior, such as licensure, peer review, and malpractice litigation, were inadequate to gauge the performance of the emerging corporate sector. Efforts to monitor individual performance failed to account for institutional performance; efforts to achieve the best outcomes for individual patients led to large disparities in diagnosis and treatment.[6]

Just as state medical boards struggled for years to devise a proper formula to evaluate physicians' performance, so corporate providers searched for appropriate criteria to judge their own performance. The essential difference was that HMOs had not taken the Hippocratic Oath. Proponents of managed care viewed the provision of medical services from the standpoint of enrolled populations, not individual patients.[7] Free to follow their own path, proponents supported a different model of medicine that rested on "systematic, replicable, statistical research," rather than "internalized, intuitive professional judgments."[8] Science-based medicine, they asserted, could provide sufficient criteria for choosing among health plans, physicians, and treatment regimens. Accumulating data on medical outcomes in large patient populations supported the development of practice profiles or report cards that allowed comparison among managed-care organizations.[9]

But there was more to evaluating medical practice than furnishing information to consumers about different health plans. Science-based medicine laid the foundation for a corporate culture that regulated physician performance.[10] Just as codes of ethics and disciplinary rules were tools of the professional order, so treatment protocols and practice guidelines were tools of the new corporate regime. According to health economist Alain Enthoven, a high-quality organization "monitors physicians' performance with accurate data on clinical outcomes and patient satisfaction. It develops ways to help physicians improve. It adjusts physicians' tasks to their current competencies. And it is able and willing to take corrective action if performance turns poor or physicians become impaired."[11]

This corporate environment that Enthoven described eschewed a role for outsiders, particularly government. Claiming that governments worked by "coercion and punishment," Enthoven asserted that they hindered quality improvement and the ability of managed-care organizations to adjust to market demands. Governments' role, he stated, was to aid in developing appropriate criteria for quality assessment and performance and to report these results to purchasers and consumers of medical services.[12] The federal government, a strong supporter of efforts to control costs, basically adopted the approach of Enthoven and of other economists. Not only did the Agency for Health Care Policy and Research pursue medical outcomes to advance treatment protocols, but peer review organizations shifted their focus from discipline to quality improvement. According to the OIG's Mark Yessian, the move toward continuous quality improvement was the reason PROs sanctioned so few physicians.[13] Unless health-care fraud was at issue, the federal government rarely took punitive action.

In truth, CQI's roots lay outside the health-care industry. For years, Japanese and some American manufacturers had applied the technique to increase productivity among their workers. The idea, in essence, was that

efforts to improve work processes rather than solve problems would promote teamwork and unity. Searching for outliers, or bad apples, was counterproductive. Fear of discovery encouraged workers to defend themselves,
as opposed to taking corrective action.[14] To many physicians, this approach
was enticing. They welcomed collegial efforts to enhance performance.[15]
But CQI operated within an institutional, not a professional, framework.
It stressed the solving of problems through an interdisciplinary perspective
and was a significant "departure from the culture of fee-for-service solo
practice."[16] CQI was further proof that the new corporate culture reduced
the ability of professions to protect their turf.

Corporate medicine and the economic model that it promoted threatened to dismantle the existing regulatory structure that included state medical boards. Boards were now out of step in that they punished physicians
for a variety of transgressions. The doyens of CQI suggested that some government regulation was necessary, but they limited it to the most serious
offenders, not those who required monitoring and education to improve
their performance.[17] Efforts of boards to regulate the quality of medical care
through disciplinary actions seemed at cross-purposes with the approach of
CQI. Restricting the role of government in policing the emerging health-
care system made boards gatekeepers and little more.

Corporate leaders also opposed attempts by boards to monitor the utilization review activities of HMOs. Although state laws gave boards the
power to regulate the practice of medicine, HMOs argued that boards had
no authority over their internal affairs. This assertion had far-reaching implications, particularly since efforts to standardize medical practice through
treatment protocols and similar procedures fragmented responsibility for
patient care. By requiring approval of treatment decisions before providing insurance coverage, HMOs could override examining physicians. If
managed-care organizations successfully prevented boards from scrutiniz-
ing patient-care decisions of their medical personnel, then the future of state
medical boards in the emerging health-care system appeared rather dim.

Another problem for boards was growing emphasis on technology, teamwork, and use of paraprofessional workers to reduce costs and promote quality. Some physicians, like Lawrence Weed, recognized these trends and called
for sweeping changes in the nature of medical decision making. Weed observed that the practice of medicine had become so complex that it had outpaced the capacity of individual physicians to integrate new information
and to manage a diverse patient population. Specialization, he argued, was
not the answer because specialists often overlooked diagnostic and man-

agement options outside their narrow fields. The failure of physicians to rely on external aids and involve their patients in treatment decisions, according to Weed, had contributed to excessive costs for medical care and to an epidemic of medical injury.[18]

The Pew Health Profession's Commission echoed Weed's call for the reform of medical practice. Among its recommendations were the "redesign" of the workforce to favor primary care, downsizing or "right-sizing" the health-care professions, and revising the tools of professional accountability. These market-driven changes that the commission envisioned struck at the heart of professional sovereignty. As part of the old power structure, state medical boards fared poorly in the commission's analysis. Although limitations on scope of practice were of primary concern, the commission also reaffirmed the perception that physician-controlled boards were "largely unaccountable to the public they served."[19]

The Pew Commission's assertion foretold the uphill battle boards faced for credibility in the new corporate order. Boards were rarely, if ever, mentioned by those searching for ways to hold managed-care organizations accountable for poor performance.[20] Many, of course, justifiably believed that the focus of boards on physician licensure and discipline made them poor candidates for policing institutional providers.[21] But those who argued that boards were unsuited to the task because of lapses in performance or adherence to outmoded norms and ethics overlooked the progress that boards had made over the past fifteen years and their legitimate role in regulating medical practice, however conceived. Public concerns about organized medicine when it controlled health care now applied to corporate medicine. As Schattschneider keenly observed, "organization is itself a mobilization of bias in preparation for action."[22] Proponents of corporate medicine were also capable of creating a self-governing order that served their interests.

Building a New Regulatory Framework

Corporate domination of American medicine was a gradual process that began long before the appearance of powerful HMOs in the 1980s and 1990s. Changes in American society predisposed the development of institutions that supported for-profit medicine, just as they did those that bolstered the medical profession. Paul Starr's study of organized medicine demonstrated that cultural authority was "antecedent to action."[23] Medical schools, hospitals, medical societies, and medical boards did not appear overnight. Broad social, economic, and political forces preceded them, including industrialization, urbanization, and specialization. Physicians' claim to superior knowledge and expertise sustained institutions that converted cultural authority into professional dominance.

The rise of corporate medicine also rested on broad currents in American society that undermined the professional order. Some called it the "deprofessionalization," others the "proletarianization," of the medical workforce. Marie Haug, the principal proponent of deprofessionalization, pointed to trends that had reduced the "knowledge gap" between physicians and consumers, such as rising levels of education, greater availability of information through use of computers, increasing complexity of medical practice, and a growing number of paraprofessional workers. Individual physicians no longer monopolized a specific body of knowledge, Haug asserted. Consumers collaborated with physicians in their care and treatment.[24]

Proponents of the proletarianization thesis also identified societal trends supporting their position that capitalist expansion had caused a decline in professional autonomy.[25] These trends included corporate consolidation of the health-care industry, increased numbers of salaried physicians working in large organizations, and the rise of intermediaries who dictated the terms of the doctor-patient relationship. Managed-care organizations embodied these trends, bolstering the notion that large organizations, not consumers, were the central players in the emerging system.

However characterized, corporate medicine gained a foothold because government and physicians failed to control costs.[26] During the 1970s policy makers turned to market competition as the mechanism for containing costs and allocating services. They also reversed prior trends through deregulation of highly regulated industries. Deregulation typically involved relaxation of government standards, making it more profitable for companies to compete. This was the case in transportation where economists claimed laws stifled market competition, but not in health care where the medical profession regulated entry, price, and delivery of services. To overcome the institutional and legal barriers that medicine had erected, the federal government passed laws to protect the development of corporate medicine and authorized federal agencies to break up the medical monopoly. Whereas the former self-governing order opposed lay control over professional judgment, commercial exploitation of medical practice, and conflicting professional loyalties, the emerging regulatory framework encouraged managerial oversight, market competition, and integration of insurance and provider systems.

Managed-care organizations benefited from the widening scope of conflict in health care. Behind the shift in power from providers to payers of medical services was a corresponding shift from local to national and from decentralized to centralized controls. Pressures to increase profits as well as reduce costs fueled the effort. As Mark Peterson observed, "a decentralized system with myriad local- or state-based carriers and providers is being supplanted by giant regional and national enterprises in search of a profit."[27] Many predicted continued integration of group practices, insurers, hospitals, and HMOs, and some even suggested that only a handful of conglomerates eventually would assume control of the entire system.[28]

If true, this had serious implications for the future regulation of the practice of medicine. Because HMOs created financial incentives to underserve, the dilemma for physicians was potentially profound. Physicians' fiduciary duty to their patients conflicted with the financial arrangements that managed care imposed. Providers and payers did not play by the same rules. Efforts by HMOs to retain premium dollars gave rise to multiple compensation schemes, including capitation, pay withholds, bonuses, and penalties, that forced physicians to share in the risk of treating sick patients. According to Deborah Stone, many physicians resented sick patients because of the drain on their income.[29] Although the economic model looked attractive on paper, market-based incentives skewed relations among physicians and their patients. Physicians required guidance in discerning conflicts of interest, and consumers required protection from the excesses of managed care. Science-based medicine and quality improvement were welcome additions, but oversight of managed-care plans was needed to correct the imbalance.[30]

The Place of Boards in the New Corporate Order

This study has viewed the struggle for power in American medicine as largely the attempt by special interests to capture the regulatory apparatus of government.[31] So long as organized medicine dominated the health-care industry, government worked to its benefit. Courts, legislatures, and state medical boards largely sanctioned the policies of the medical profession. As political scientist Corinne Gilb observed when writing in the 1960s, "government, for the stronger professional associations, is a continuum, a matter of continual interaction between private and public governments."[32] Boards were part of this continuum.

Those who controlled the regulatory apparatus often succeeded in keeping conflict private. For weaker interests to prevail, they had to politicize the struggle by widening the scope of conflict. In the case of state medical boards, consumer groups, the media, and malpractice insurers persuaded courts, state agencies, and state legislatures to enhance medical discipline for public protection. But it took much more to alter old patterns. The changing contours of medical discipline reflected an ideological struggle between the profession of medicine and the business of medicine. In this power struggle, government took center stage because of the enormous costs of health care. Government's solution to the problem of rising costs, market competition in the health-care sector, precipitated the entry of new forces, as well as the realignment of old ones.

Corporate integration of the health-care industry had distinct advantages over traditional fee-for-service medicine, among them better coordination of medical services, the development of practice guidelines, enhanced accountability, and cost savings. There was no turning back. Recognizing the situation, physicians responded through closer oversight of their colleagues. Medical groups collected information on practice patterns of individual physicians.[33] Hospitals and professional associations incorporated IPPs, formal peer review, and continuous quality improvement. The AMA expanded existing databases and formulated new ones to increase physician accountability.[34] The bureaucratization of medical practice, characterized by hierarchy, formality, and standardized procedures, occurred at all levels in all professional institutions.

State medical boards, for their part, sought to survive by improving case management and reporting procedures. For a market-oriented approach to succeed, consumers needed reliable information based on quality and cost to aid in choosing among providers. Boards were key to quality control: they were the primary mechanisms for disciplining physicians for substandard care, drug abuse, sexual misconduct, and a variety of other offenses. Moreover, they were the only ones responsible for telling the public about it. No other entity seemed interested in ridding the medical profession of the poor practitioners. As James Winn, executive vice president of the Federation of State Medical Boards, observed, "corporations aren't very good about exposing themselves to potential litigation or bad publicity. If they've got a bad doctor, they're going to quietly show him the door. They're not going to tell the medical boards about it."[35]

Attempts to reform the disciplinary process by consolidating state licensing boards, as the Pew Commission suggested, would likely fail in the current climate and in the foreseeable future. State medical societies, a potent force in state politics, have historically resisted measures designed to upset the status quo. State medical boards are also in a better position to protect their power base and membership. Their staffs have grown considerably during the 1990s, they have established regional and national alliances, and they have become information centers for government, consumers, hospitals, and managed-care entities. Indeed, state medical boards have distanced themselves from other licensing boards. Most are self-funded entities, able to function on their own. Tying them to other government agencies might rekindle old budgetary constraints.

For several reasons, boards' overall responsibility for public protection is expanding, not contracting, in a managed-care environment. Responsibility for health policy and planning devolved to the states after Congress failed to enact the Clinton administration's proposed model for health-care reform.[36] Now more than ever, states need boards to police the practice of medicine. While old problems persist, new ones emerge. The conversion to for-profit medicine has increased opportunities for fraud and abuse. Reliance on low-cost providers has led to some questionable medical practices. Financial incentives to underutilize medical services have raised concerns about substandard care.

In 1994 the General Accounting Office estimated that as much as 10 percent of total health-care costs were lost to fraud and abuse each year.[37] Federal efforts to curtail the problem led to the enactment of laws prohibiting physicians from soliciting, offering, or receiving kickbacks, bribes, or rebates as well as those prohibiting physicians from referring patients to ancillary health-care facilities in which they had an ownership interest.[38] Passage of the Health Insurance Portability and Accountability Act in 1996 expanded federal oversight in this area.[39] The new law called for closer coordination among federal, state, and local authorities and the formation of another federal database to track fraud and abuse activities. The amount and type of information that federal authorities required from state medical boards under the new law was greater than in the past.[40]

For-profit medicine also advanced trends toward alternative care. To be sure, conventional medicine did not have all the answers. Many patients who suffered from chronic pain or disease turned to alternative therapies when conventional ones failed. As in the past, nonphysician providers, such as chiropractors, promised relief from some symptoms. But unlike in the past, alternative therapies received support from the new status quo. In 1996 the Oxford Health Plans, a major HMO, offered coverage for nontraditional care, including acupuncture, chiropractic, and naturopathy (*New York Times*, 13 Nov. 1996). Maintaining customer satisfaction was a reason for an expanded list of providers, but some HMOs viewed alternative medicine as an opportunity for cost savings on conventional care. Boards monitored these developments closely, poised to take action should physicians venture too far.[41]

Few of these activities were particularly controversial. The architects of the emerging order agreed that it would be a mistake to abandon surveillance and discipline of "the truly avaricious and the dangerously incompetent."[42] But boards were not content to stand on the sidelines, disciplining the castoffs from managed-care organizations. Inspired by their leaders, many signaled their intentions to become central players in the quality assurance debate.[43] Regulating the utilization review activities of HMOs as in Arizona was one example; monitoring quality assurance programs of hospitals and other health-care facilities as in Massachusetts was another. Some also suggested that boards promote policies to bolster the status of salaried physicians.[44]

Boards faced many obstacles in these new endeavors, including the capacity for such initiatives. According to Mark Yessian, identifying patterns of substandard care "is the most difficult challenge, for it pushes boards into new directions involving the extensive examination of medical records, the use of statistical sampling and analysis, and the interpretation of evolving medical practice guidelines."[45] HMOs viewed boards as infringing on their decisions. Others suggested that boards were not right for the job because they focused on individuals, not integrated systems.[46] At the heart of the matter was the struggle for control of the evolving regulatory structure. Managed care sought to keep boards at bay. Boards sought to expand their authority.

If not boards, then who? What other state agencies existed to curb the abuses of managed care? The answer was that there really were none, despite all the rhetoric. State insurance departments seemed likely candidates because they regulated the insurance industry, but studies showed that their ability to monitor quality was quite limited.[47] Faced with a consumer backlash against managed care, thirty-seven states passed protective legislation in 1996, ranging from minimum hospital stays for maternity patients to specific quality assurance standards.[48] Although few health-care experts supported such legislation, arguing that these laws stifled growth and creativity in the private sector, the size and scale of the undertaking signaled widespread discontent.[49] For many Americans, doctor-patient relationships and community hospitals symbolized a health-care system devoted to compassion and altruism.[50] They perceived that managed-care organizations undermined these core values and institutions.

State medical boards offered an effective check on the emerging health-care industry. Although many dismissed boards as candidates for public protection because of their past and continuing affiliation with organized medicine, protecting the public required balancing norms and values of business and of profession. One way to achieve this balance was to secure a role for the medical profession in the ongoing struggle. Boards provided the medical profession with an important voice in the governing process.

For many years political scientists have debated the extent to which responsiveness to political authority should supersede the norms and ethics of professionals working for American government. Fueling the debate were political initiatives, such as those in the area of family planning and abortion, that compromised professional ideals. Although politicians often voiced their concern that bureaucrats threatened majority will, others expressed the belief that, in certain instances, professional standards and values should have priority. As political scientist Francis Rourke proclaimed, "The public itself benefits from having professionals within bureaucracy speak out strongly against policies that violate the ethical or technical canons of their own calling, since these canons are often designed to advance and protect the public interest, and are not solely intended to protect the interests of the professional groups themselves."[51]

Just as professional values acted as checks on political authority, so they also protected the public from the excesses of managed care. Efforts by HMOs to maximize profits by introducing incentives to underutilize medical services tested the allegiance of physicians to their patients. Disciplinary rules and professional ethics governing doctor-patient relations potentially conflicted with corporate norms of behavior. Whether corporate enterprise develops adequate mechanisms to ensure quality in the face of economic incentives to cut costs and maximize profits remains to be seen. The current challenge to state medical boards is maintaining professional accountability within a diffused corporate hierarchy driven by multiprofessionals and profit motives.

Introduction

1. Throughout this book, I use the term *state medical boards* generically to include those licensing and disciplinary bodies that are members of the Federation of State Medical Boards of the United States, Inc. Membership in the federation has fluctuated since its founding in 1912. As of 1997, the federation's membership totaled sixty-eight boards as follows: fifty-four allopathic boards from each of the fifty states, the District of Columbia, Puerto Rico, Guam, and the Virgin Islands, and fourteen osteopathic boards from the states of Arizona, California, Florida, Maine, Michigan, Nevada, New Mexico, Oklahoma, Pennsylvania, Tennessee, Utah, Vermont, Washington, and West Virginia.

2. For the most part, physician discipline, not licensure, has captured the headlines. One notable exception concerned the licensure of foreign medical graduates (FMGs), a problem that surfaced in the early 1980s following the establishment of proprietary medical schools in the Caribbean, the distribution of fake medical degrees from some of these schools, and cheating scandals on exams administered to FMGs. In response, boards tightened their standards for licensure of FMGs through testing, graduate medical education, and more comprehensive screening of candidates. See Department of Health and Human Services, Office of the Inspector General (hereafter DHHS, OIG), *Medical Licensure and Discipline: An Overview* (Boston: Office of Evaluation and Inspections, 1986), 1–10.

By focusing on discipline, I do not mean to overlook the role of state medical boards in licensing physicians or the way in which licensing and discipline are intertwined. In the early chapters, I discuss why licensing, not discipline, was the central concern of boards. I also link public pressures to discipline physicians in the 1970s and 1980s to federal incentives to increase the number of practitioners.

3. Cf. Deborah A. Stone, "The Doctor as Businessman: The Changing Politics of a Cultural Icon," *Journal of Health Politics, Policy, and Law* 22 (Apr. 1997): 537–41; Ezekial J. Emanuel and Linda L. Emanuel, "Preserving Community in Health Care," *Journal of Health Politics, Policy, and Law* 22 (Feb. 1997): 154–55.

4. Raymond McKeown, *Report of the Medical Disciplinary Committee to the Board of Trustees* (Chicago: American Medical Association, 1961), 46, 55 (emphasis in original). State and local (county) medical societies are components of the American Medical Association, an umbrella organization that also unites specialty medical societies, hospital medical staffs, and medical schools. All organizational components are functionally independent of the AMA, hence the designation "Federation of Medicine." I use the term *organized medicine* to describe the AMA and its component organizations. I use the terms *professional associations* and *medical societies* interchangeably when referring to state and local medical societies.

5. Robert C. Derbyshire, "How Effective Is Medical Self-regulation?" *Law and Human Behavior* 7, nos. 2/3 (1983): 197. See also Derbyshire's earlier study on which

these calculations are based: *Medical Licensure and Discipline in the United States* (Baltimore: Johns Hopkins Press, 1969), 76–90.

6. Derbyshire, "Medical Self-regulation," 197.

7. Department of Health, Education, and Welfare, *Report on Licensure and Related Health Personnel Credentialing,* DHEW Publication no. (HSM)72-11 (Washington, D.C., 1971), 33. Follow-up studies include Department of Health, Education, and Welfare, *Developments in Health Manpower Licensure,* DHEW Publication no.(HRA) 74-3101 (Washington, D.C., 1973) and Department of Health, Education, and Welfare, *Credentialing Health Manpower,* DHEW Publication no.(OS)77-50057 (Washington, D.C., 1977).

8. Frank P. Grad and Noelia Marti, *Physicians' Licensure and Discipline* (Dobbs Ferry, N.Y.: Oceana Publications, 1979).

9. Andrew K. Dolan and Nicole D. Urban, "The Determinants of the Effectiveness of Medical Disciplinary Boards: 1960–1977," *Law and Human Behavior* 7, nos. 2/3 (1983): 215–16.

10. Sidney M. Wolfe, Henry Bergman, and George Silver, *Medical Malpractice: The Need for Disciplinary Reform, Not Tort Reform,* (Washington, D.C.: Public Citizen Health Research Group, 1985). The Association of Trial Lawyers of America adopted a similar position. See *Wichita Business Journal,* 4 Apr. 1988; American Medical Association, "Report of the Special Task Force on Professional Liability and Insurance and the Advisory Panel on Professional Liability," *JAMA* 257 (13 Feb. 1987): 810–11; Professional Liability Commentary, "Two Views on the Malpractice Insurance Crisis," *Journal of the Medical Society of New Jersey* 82 (Sept. 1985): 710–14.

11. American Medical Association, "Report of the Special Task Force on Professional Liability," 810–12; Congress, House of Representatives, Committee on Energy and Commerce, *The Health Care Quality Improvement Act of 1986: Hearing before the Subcommittee on Health and the Environment* (statement of James S. Todd, M.D., senior deputy executive vice president of the AMA), 99th Cong., 2d session, 18 Mar. 1986, 86; *New York Times,* 2 Sept. 1985.

12. Otis R. Bowen, "Congressional Testimony on Senate Bill S. 1804," *JAMA* 257 (13 Feb. 1987): 816–18.

13. Ingrid VanTuinen, Phyllis McCarthy, and Sidney Wolfe, *Questionable Doctors* (Washington, D.C.: Public Citizen Health Research Group, 1991).

14. Department of Health and Human Services, Office of the Inspector General, *The Peer Review Organizations and State Medical Boards: A Vital Link* (Boston: Office of Evaluation and Inspections, 1993), 1.

15. Ibid. See also David A. Swankin and Debi H. Tucker, *Information Exchange between Peer Review Organizations and Medical Licensing Boards: Report on 50 State Survey* (Washington, D.C.: Citizen Advocacy Center, 1992), 2–7.

16. Panel Discussion on Peer Review (Lecture by Otto C. Page, M.D.), *Maryland State Medical Journal* (Jan. 1973): 42.

17. Cf. George Anders, *Health against Wealth: HMOs and the Breakdown of Medical Trust* (Boston: Houghton Mifflin, 1996), 183, 215–17, 230–31.

18. Cf. Gail R. Wilensky, "Promoting Quality: A Public Policy View," *Health Affairs* 16 (May/June 1997): 80.

19. Mark R. Yessian, "State Medical Boards and Quality Assurance," *Federation Bulletin* 79 (Sept. 1992): 126–35.

20. Bernadette Lane, executive director, Baltimore City Medical Society, interview by author, 11 Apr. 1995; Sidney Wolfe et al., *Questionable Doctors* (Washington, D.C.: Public Citizen Health Research Group, 1993), ix–x; congressional hearings on the Health Care Quality Improvement Act of 1986 (testimony of Dale G. Breaden, associate executive vice president, Federation of State Medical Boards), 389.

21. Sidney Wolfe et al., *Questionable Doctors* (Washington, D.C.: Public Citizen Health Research Group, 1996), 8.

22. Ibid., 13.

23. Derbyshire, "Medical Self-regulation," 198.

24. Wolfe et al., *Questionable Doctors* (1996), 23.

25. Ibid., 19–20.

26. Gwen Andrew and Harold Sauer, "Do Boards of Medicine Really Matter? The Future of Professional Regulation," *Federation Bulletin* 83, no. 4 (1996): 234–35.

27. Dale G. Breaden and Bryant L. Galusha, *Official 1985 Federation Summary of Reported Disciplinary Actions* (Fort Worth, Tex.: Federation of State Medical Boards, 1986), 300–301.

28. Massachusetts is the first state to release information on malpractice actions and hospital discipline. See Alexander F. Fleming, "Massachusetts Physician Profiles," *Federation Bulletin* 84, no. 1 (1997): 9. State medical societies often oppose such efforts, as in Maryland (*Baltimore Sun,* 19 Dec. 1996).

29. Mark A. Peterson, "Health Care into the Next Century," *Journal of Health Politics, Policy and Law* 22 (Apr. 1997): 297.

30. The current emphasis in both the public and private sectors is on quality improvement, not quality oversight. See Mark R. Yessian, "Quality of Care Cases: Issues of Competence and Substandard Care," Keynote Speaker, annual meeting of the Federation of State Medical Boards, Apr. 1994; Timothy Jost, "Health System Reform: Forward or Backward with Quality Oversight?" *JAMA* 271 (18 May 1994): 1508–11.

31. Cf. John P. Seward, "Restoring the Ethical Balance in Health Care," *Health Affairs* 16 (May/June 1997): 195–97; Carol C. Nadelson, "Emerging Issues in Medical Ethics," *British Journal of Psychiatry* 158 (1991): 9–16.

32. See Stone, "Doctor as Businessman," 551.

33. Seward, "Restoring the Ethical Balance," 196–97.

34. E. E. Schattschneider, *The Semisovereign People: A Realist's View of Democracy in America* (New York: Holt, Rinehart and Winston, 1960; reprint, Hinsdale, Ill.: Dryden Press, 1975), 2 (emphasis in original); page references are to reprint edition.

35. Ibid., 7.

36. Cf. Jeffrey L. Berlant, *Profession and Monopoly: A Study of Medicine in the*

United States and Great Britain (Berkeley: University of California Press, 1975); Peri Rosenfeld, "Protecting the Public or Promoting the Profession: A Sociological History of Medical Licensing Law, 1880–1910" (Ph.D. dissertation, State University of New York at Stony Brook, 1984).

37. W. Richard Scott, "Health Care Organizations in the 1980's: The Convergence of Public and Professional Control Systems," in *Organizational Environments: Ritual and Rationality*, ed. John W. Meyer and W. Richard Scott (Newbury Park, Calif.: Sage Publications, 1992), 101.

38. Schattschneider, *Semisovereign People*, 11.

39. Richard P. Kusserow, Elisabeth A. Handley, and Mark R. Yessian, "An Overview of State Medical Discipline," *JAMA* 257 (13 Feb. 1987): 822.

40. Schattschneider, *Semisovereign People*, 119.

41. Paul Starr, *The Social Transformation of American Medicine* (New York: Basic Books, 1982), 5.

42. Paul J. Feldstein, *Health Policy Issues: An Economic Perspective on Health Reform* (Ann Arbor, Mich.: AUPHA Press/Health Administration Press, 1994), 234–36.

43. Starr, *Social Transformation*, 396.

44. Schattschneider, *Semisovereign People*, 72. Cf. Wilensky, "Promoting Quality."

45. Trish Riley, "The Role of States in Accountability for Quality," *Health Affairs* 16 (May/June 1997): 41–43.

46. George R. Buck, *A Guide to the Essentials Of a Modern Medical Practice Act* (Fort Worth, Tex.: Federation of State Medical Boards, 1956).

47. See Melvin E. Sigel, M.D., *Elements of a Modern State Medical Board: A Proposal* (Fort Worth, Tex.: Federation of State Medical Boards, 1989), 8–9.

48. Robert E. Porter, "Report of the American Medical Association and the Federation of State Medical Boards: Ethics and Quality of Care," *Federation Bulletin* 82, no. 2 (1995), 91.

Chapter 1. The Professional Order

1. See, e.g., Schattschneider, *Semisovereign People*, 116.

2. Federal government involvement in health care actually began in 1946 when Congress passed the Hospital Survey and Construction Act (Hill-Burton). Under the Hill-Burton program, the federal government subsidized the construction of public health-care facilities, primarily general community hospitals. See Theodore R. Marmor, *Understanding Health Care Reform* (New Haven: Yale University Press, 1994), 57.

3. Professional associations, that is, state and local medical societies, impose private sanctions when they expel, suspend, or deny membership status. Private sanctions may also include group boycotts or other forms of deterrence.

State medical boards impose public sanctions when they revoke, suspend, reprimand, or issue a public order in any way limiting or restricting a license. Rather than taking formal action, state boards may proceed informally by meeting with licensees to discuss possible misconduct. This may end the matter or result in an informal letter of reprimand, a letter of admonishment, or a letter to cease and desist from offensive activities.

Credentialing decisions involve a physician's qualifications for affiliation with a hospital or related institution. Educational background, licensing, and specialty board certification are central components of the credentialing process.

4. Cf. John C. Burnham, "American Medicine's Golden Age: What Happened to It?" *Science* 215 (Mar. 1982): 1476–78; Troyen A. Brennan, *Just Doctoring* (Berkeley: University of California Press, 1991), 16–49.

5. AMA, *Report of the Medical Disciplinary Committee* (1961), 13–14.

6. Raymond McKeown, "Present Status of Medical Discipline," *Federation Bulletin* 48 (1961): 141.

7. George Rosen, *The Structure of American Medical Practice, 1875–1941* (Philadelphia: University of Pennsylvania Press, 1983), 20–35; James G. Burrow, *Organized Medicine in the Progressive Era: The Move toward Monopoly* (Baltimore: Johns Hopkins University Press, 1977), 15.

8. Richard Harrison Shryock, *Medical Licensing in America, 1650–1965* (Baltimore: Johns Hopkins Press, 1967), 28.

9. Allopaths used conventional means, such as surgery or concentrated doses of drugs, to combat disease. Sectarians, on the other hand, treated disease in ways which allopaths argued had little or no scientific basis. Today most of these so-called irregular techniques fall into the category of alternative medicine. When using the term *physician,* I mean allopath or "regular" practitioner of medicine.

10. Burrow, *Organized Medicine in the Progressive Era,* 57.

11. Shryock, *Medical Licensing in America,* 29.

12. Rosen, *Structure of American Medical Practice,* 24.

13. See Starr, *Social Transformation,* 92 (emphasis in original).

14. A. D. Bevan, "Report of the Council on Medical Education and Hospitals," *JAMA* 76 (11 June 1921): 1677; Starr, *Social Transformation,* 102.

15. James A. Johnson and Walter J. Jones, *The American Medical Association and Organized Medicine* (New York: Garland Publishing, 1993), 19.

16. Shryock, *Medical Licensing in America,* 48.

17. Burrow, *Organized Medicine in Progressive Era,* 58–59.

18. Ibid., 58; Council on Medical Education (hereafter CME) Report (11 June 1921), 1677.

19. Starr, *Social Transformation,* 107.

20. Scholle v. State, 90 Md. 729 (1900).

21. The Regents Case, 9 Gill & J. 365, 387–90 (Md. 1836).

22. Act of 1838, ch. 281.

23. John C. French, *A Brief History of the Medical and Chirurgical Faculty of Maryland* (Baltimore: Waverly Press, 1949), 17.

24. Act of 1892, ch. 269. The Maryland legislature enacted a law in 1867 establishing a licensing scheme but repealed it one year later. The legislature passed

another licensing law in 1888, which it modified by an act in 1892. The 1892 act gave Med Chi licensing authority.

25. Reddick v. State, 130 A.2d 762 (Md. 1957).

26. Dent v. State of West Virginia, 129 U.S. 114 (1888).

27. Dent, 129 U.S. at 123.

28. Kermit L. Hall, *The Magic Mirror* (New York: Oxford University Press, 1989), 235.

29. Dent, 129 U.S. at 122–23.

30. Scholle, 90 Md. at 740. See also Dent, 129 U.S. at 114.

31. Report of the Board of Medical Examiners of Maryland to the Medical and Chirurgical Faculty, 31 Dec. 1923, Maryland State Archives.

32. Scholle, 90 Md. at 741–44; Wilkins v. State, 113 Ind. 514 (1888); Ex parte McNulty, 77 Cal. 164 (1888); Iowa Med. As. v. Schrader, 87 Iowa 659 (1893).

33. Before the 1970s many courts, including the Supreme Court, considered cases challenging license revocation on procedural due process grounds including right to notice and hearing. State of Missouri ex rel. Hurwitz v. North et al., Board of Health of the State of Missouri, 271 U.S. 40 (1925). See Law Division of the AMA, *Disciplinary Digest* (Chicago: American Medical Association, 1967); "Rights as to Notice and Hearing in Proceeding to Revoke or Suspend License to Practice Medicine," 10 ALR 5th 1 (Rochester: Lawyers Cooperative Publishing, 1993). The Supreme Court first entertained equal protection challenges to board composition in *Gibson v. Berryhill,* 411 U.S. 564 (1973) and in *Freidman v. Rogers,* 440 U.S. 1 (1979). In *Freidman,* the Court upheld a law requiring that a majority of the members of the Texas Optometry Board be selected from the Texas Optometric Association.

34. Maryland Medical Practice Act (1902) ch. 612, sec. 65. Some states used different language to capture certain "generic offenses." "Manifest incapacity," for instance, related to mental or physical disability from drug or alcohol abuse. "Infamous conduct" encompassed crimes involving moral turpitude. See Law Division of the AMA, *Disciplinary Digest,* 15–16. Some early boards, among them that of Illinois in 1933 and the Board of Health of the Territory of Hawaii in 1931, charged physicians with "gross carelessness," but this was atypical.

35. Constitution, Bylaws, and Fee Table of the Medical and Chirurgical Faculty of the State of Maryland, 23 Mar. 1875, Special Collections, Medical and Chirurgical Faculty Library, Baltimore.

36. Oliver Garceau, *The Political Life of the American Medical Association* (Cambridge, Mass.: Harvard University Press, 1941), 106; Eugene Fontelroy Cordell, *The Medical Annals of Maryland, 1799–1899* (Baltimore: Medical and Chirurgical Faculty, 1903), 77, 119, 144, 170.

37. A. M. Carr-Saunders and P. A. Wilson, *The Professions* (Oxford: Clarendon Press, 1933), 398–401.

38. John M. Dodson, "Report of the Council on Medical Education," *JAMA* 72 (14 June 1919): 1752–53.

39. CME Report (14 June 1919), 1752.

40. Starr, *Social Transformation,* 120–21.

41. Editorial, "Closing the Back Doors to Medical Licensure," *JAMA* 89 (20 Aug. 1927): 625.

42. James S. Roberts, Jack G. Coale, and Robert R. Redman, "A History of the Joint Commission on Accreditation of Hospitals," *JAMA* 258 (21 Aug. 1987): 936–38.

43. Ibid., 938–40.

44. CME Report (11 June 1921), 1672–73.

45. Garceau, *Political Life of the AMA,* 50–57.

46. Shryock, *Medical Licensing in America,* 68–70. Shryock suggests either that boards were attempting "to avoid another responsibility" or that specialists "preferred to keep controls out of official hands." After reviewing CME reports and other accounts of clashes between generalists and specialists, I believe that specialty licensure was a politically charged issue that the profession could not resolve publicly without creating deep resentment among practitioners.

47. Office of General Counsel of the AMA, *Establishment and Enforcement of Standards in the Medical Profession,* 23–27; Council on Medical Education, "Physician Credentialing and Privileging," in *Proceedings of the House of Delegates of the American Medical Association* (Chicago: American Medical Association, 1993), 290–92; Maryland Hospital Education Institute, III-5.

48. Grad and Marti, *Physician's Licensure and Discipline,* 125. California was the first state to establish a standard for medical incompetence not related to illness.

49. AMA, *Report of the Medical Disciplinary Committee* (1961), 31–32; McKeown, "Present Status of Medical Discipline," 139.

50. AMA, *Report of the Medical Disciplinary Committee* (1961), 31–32.

51. Berlant, *Profession and Monopoly,* 99–115.

52. Council on Ethical and Judicial Affairs, *Code of Medical Ethics: Current Opinions with Annotations* (Chicago: American Medical Association, 1994), ix–x; Berlant, *Profession and Monopoly,* 97–98.

53. Garceau, *Political Life of the AMA,* 17.

54. Burrow, *Organized Medicine in the Progressive Era,* 65.

55. See AMA, *Disciplinary Digest,* 6; Burrow, *Organized Medicine in the Progressive Era,* 64. The terms *unprofessional conduct* or *professional misconduct* are somewhat ambiguous. Boards often used such grounds as a "catchall" where no specific ground applied. When categorizing disciplinary actions, some individuals and organizations include ethics violations under "unprofessional conduct" while others do not. Derbyshire included ethics violations under unprofessional conduct. Public Citizen lists them under "failure to comply with a professional rule." Unless otherwise indicated, I will include ethics violations under the heading *unprofessional conduct.*

56. Berlant, *Profession and Monopoly,* 65. See, generally, Starr, *Social Transformation*; Garceau, *Political Life of the AMA*; and Stanley J. Gross, *Of Foxes and Hen*

Houses: Licensing and the Healing Professions (Westport, Conn.: Greenwood Press, 1984).

57. Frank Riggall, "Do We Need a Code of Medical Ethics?" *Medical Economics* 19 (1942): 44.

58. Mark A. Hall, "Institutional Control of Physician Behavior: Legal Barriers to Health Care Cost Containment," *University of Pennsylvania Law Review* 137 (1988): 431, 488–504.

59. Starr, *Social Transformation,* 299–306.

60. American Medical Association v. U.S., 317 U.S. 519 (1943).

61. I reviewed available reports of the Board of Medical Examiners of the State of Maryland for the years 1898, 1900, 1902, 1903, 1923, 1924, 1925, 1926, 1927, and 1929. During the period these reports encompass, I discovered only one reported revocation in 1926 for a narcotics violation. Some reports indicated ongoing investigations for fee splitting and advertising. See also Derbyshire, *Medical Licensure,* 78; AMA, *Report of the Medical Disciplinary Committee* (1961), App. 3-A.

62. George E. Follansbee, "Report of the Judicial Council," *JAMA* 104 (22 June 1935): 2267.

63. The Medical Disciplinary Committee of the AMA reported in June 1961, almost thirty years after the Judicial Council's report, that a few state societies "in recent years" have established independent committees to hear "intra-professional disciplinary problems." Even so, the small number of reported actions suggests that medical societies rarely activated such committees. See AMA, *Report of the Medical Disciplinary Committee* (1961), App. 4.

64. The minutes of the Board of Medical Examiners of the State of Maryland for the period 1950 to 1970 reflect numerous instances of stern warnings and letters of reprimand issued to licensees for ethical misconduct. There were clear differences between how the board handled these cases and how it handled those involving outside law enforcement agencies. In cases concerning violations of the criminal laws pertaining to narcotics or abortion, the board was more inclined to take formal disciplinary action.

65. Note, "The American Medical Association: Power, Purpose, and Politics in Organized Medicine," *Yale Law Journal* 63 (1954): 949–53.

66. Eliot Freidson, *Professional Dominance: The Social Structure of Medical Care* (New York: Atherton Press, 1970), 89, 91.

67. Starr, *Social Transformation,* 146; Rosen, *Structure of American Medical Practice,* 48.

68. Charles Perrow, "Hospitals, Technology, Structure, and Goals," in *Handbook of Organizations,* ed. James G. March (Chicago: Rand McNally, 1965), 947–52; Starr, *Social Transformation,* 177–79.

69. Starr, *Social Transformation,* 168.

70. Rosen, *Structure of American Medical Practice,* 114; Note, "Power, Purpose, and Politics," 952.

71. U.S. v. Oregon State Medical Society, 343 U.S. 326 (1952); Riggall v. Wash-

ington County Medical Society, 249 F.2d 266 (8th Cir. 1957); Speers Free Clinic and Hospital v. Cleere, 197 F.2d 125 (10th Cir. 1952).

72. Greisman v. Newcomb Hospital, 192 A.2d 817 (N.J. 1963).

73. People v. United Medical Service, Inc., 362 Ill. 442, 200 N.E. 157 (1936). The corporate practice of medicine doctrine was an extension of the prohibition on contract practice encompassing any organization offering medical care that was not owned and operated by physicians. Despite the Supreme Court's holding in American Medical Association, 317 U.S. at 519, many states subsequently passed laws prohibiting nonphysician incorporators of medical plans.

74. The seminal case holding hospitals liable for medical staff malpractice was Darling v. Charleston Community Memorial Hospital, 211 N.E.2d 253 (Ill. 1965).

75. Note, "The Corporate Practice of Medicine Doctrine: An Anachronism in the Modern Health Care Industry," *Vanderbilt Law Review* 40 (1987): 445, 467.

76. Atchison v. State, 105 A.2d 495, 497–98 (Md. 1953).

77. Georgia Medical Practice Act (1907), sec. 84–901.

78. Maryland Medical Practice Act (1908), ch. 120.

79. Long v. Metzger, 152 A. 572, 573 (Pa. 1930).

80. *Words & Phrases,* "Practice of Medicine" (St. Paul: West Publishing, 1971).

81. E. W. Rowe, M.D., chairman, Medical Economics Committee, Nebraska State Medical Association, to R. T. Shackelford, M.D., 1 Oct. 1941, letter and accompanying "A Study of General Practice Acts," Special Collections, Medical and Chirurgical Faculty Library, Baltimore.

82. Osteopathy is "a system of treatment based on the theory that diseases are chiefly due to deranged mechanism of the bones, nerves, blood vessels, and other tissues, and can be remedied by manipulation of these parts." See Georgia Ass'n of Osteopathic Physicians & Surgeons v. Allen, 112 F.2d 52 (5th Cir. 1940), quoting from Webster's *New International Dictionary.* See also *Words & Phrases,* "Practice of Medicine," 329.

83. Chiropractic is "a drugless system of health care based on the principle that interference with the transmission of nerve impulses may cause disease. 'Practice chiropractic' includes the diagnosing and location of misaligned or displaced vertebrae and, through the manual manipulation and adjustment of the spine and other skeletal structures, treating disorders of the human body," Md. Ann. Code, *Health Occupations* (1994 repl. vol.), sec. 3-101. See also *Words & Phrases,* "Practice of Medicine," 322.

84. Study of General Practice Acts (1941).

85. CME Report (14 June 1919), 1754.

86. Charles B. Pinkham, "The Chiropractic Problem," *JAMA* 76 (2 Apr. 1921): 938.

87. Report of the Board of Medical Examiners of Maryland to the Medical and Chirurgical Faculty, 31 Dec. 1928, Maryland State Archives.

88. Andrew Abbott, *The System of Professions: An Essay on the Division of Expert Labor* (Chicago: University of Chicago Press, 1988), 77.

89. Pinkham, "Chiropractic Problem," 938.

90. Long, 152 A. at 572; State Board of Medical Examiners v. De Baun, 147 A. 744, 745 (N.J. 1929); State v. Henry 97 N.E. 2d 487, 490 (Ind. 1951).

91. "Chiropractic: Its Cause and Cure," *Medical Economics* 19 (1942): 42.

92. Report of the Board of Medical Examiners of Maryland, 31 Dec. 1928.

93. Beverungen v. Briele, 333 A.2d 664 (Md. 1975).

94. "Chiropractic: Its Cause and Cure," 42.

95. Ibid., 42–43.

96. Report of the Board of Medical Examiners of Maryland, 31 Dec. 1928.

97. Derbyshire, *Medical Licensure,* 118–21.

98. Ibid., 128. But see Pinkham, "Chiropractic Problem," 74. Writing twenty-five years before Derbyshire, Pinkham asserted that "nearly 70 percent" of chiropractors taking the basic science examination "flunk[ed]," and that basic science laws were having the desired effect in states such as Kansas.

99. Wilk v. American Medical Ass'n, 895 F.2d 352 (7th Cir. 1990); Chiropractic Coop. Ass'n v. AMA, 867 F.2d 270 (6th Cir. 1989).

100. Eliot Freidson, *Profession of Medicine: A Study of the Sociology of Applied Knowledge* (New York: Dodd, Mead, 1973; Afterword, 1988), 384.

101. E.g., Laws of Maryland 1957, ch. 29, *repealed by* Md. Ann. Code, *Health Occupations* (repl. vol. 1994), secs. 1-101-20-502.

102. Abbott, *System of Professions,* 72, 169–71.

103. Wilk, 895 F.2d at 352; Chiropractic Coop., 867 F.2d at 270.

104. Freidson, *Profession of Medicine,* 137.

105. Burnham, "American Medicine's Golden Age," 1475.

106. John H. Morton, "Politics and Medical Manpower," *Federation Bulletin* 73 (May 1986): 137.

107. Freidson, *Profession of Medicine,* 178–80; Berlant, *Profession and Monopoly,* 75–79.

108. Freidson, *Profession of Medicine,* 137–84. See also Eliot Freidson and Buford Rhea, "Processes of Control in a Company of Equals," *Social Problems* 11 (1963): 119–31.

109. Philip Wylie, "The Doctors' Conspiracy of Silence," *Medical Economics* 29 (1952): 173.

110. See Burnham, "American Medicine's Golden Age," 1475–76.

111. AMA, *Report of the Medical Disciplinary Committee* (1961), 39–40; Burnham, "American Medicine's Golden Age," 1475.

112. Interview by author of Bernadette Lane, 11 Apr. 1995.

113. Mediation Committee, "Annual Report to the House of Delegates," *Maryland State Medical Journal* (June 1970): 70.

114. AMA, *Report of the Medical Disciplinary Committee* (1961); McKeown, "Present Status of Medical Discipline," 136.

115. McKeown, "Present Status of Medical Discipline," 136.

116. AMA, *Report of the Medical Disciplinary Committee* (1961), 13. Following references to page numbers refer to this report.

117. Derbyshire, "Medical Self-regulation," 197.

118. Derbyshire, *Medical Licensure,* 77–78, 83; quotation on 87.

119. Judicial Council, "Medical Disciplinary Reports," *JAMA* 190 (1964): 122; *JAMA* 194 (1965): 124; *JAMA* 202 (1967): 165; *JAMA* 210 (1969): 1092.

120. William F. Quinn, "What We're Doing about the Bad Apples," *Medical Economics* 39 (1962): 227–38; quotation on 238.

121. McKeown, "Present Status of Medical Discipline," 141.

122. David B. Allman, M.D., "The President's Page," *JAMA* (31 May 1958): 584.

123. Charles L. Terry Jr., "The Physician as a Defendant in Discipline," in Department of Medical Ethics, *Papers on Medical Discipline* (Chicago: American Medical Association, 1962), 20, 34.

124. AMA, *Report of the Medical Disciplinary Committee* (1961), 61.

125. McKeown, "Present Status of Medical Discipline," 133.

126. AMA, *Report of the Medical Disciplinary Committee* (1961), 52.

Chapter 2. The Decline of the Professional Order

1. Before the 1970s, insurance for physician and hospital services consisted of either commercial indemnity plans or provider-controlled plans such as Blue Cross and Blue Shield. Physicians refused direct payment for services unless they controlled the plan. Starr, *Social Transformation,* 290–331.

2. Much of the information contained in figure 2.1 comes from the Federation of State Medical Boards. The federation has collected and disseminated information on formal disciplinary actions since 1915. Until the federation established its Disciplinary Data Bank in 1985, information was often incomplete. According to the federation's former executive vice president, "Few states reported regularly and those that did frequently failed to report completely, documentation was often wanting, and central storage of the collected data was primitive." Bryant L. Galusha, "Physician Disciplinary Reporting: Progress, Problems and Prospects," *Federation Bulletin* 74 (May 1987): 138. The federation issued its first annual summary of reported disciplinary actions in 1984.

3. Starr, *Social Transformation,* 367–74; Marmor, *Understanding Health Care Reform,* 57–61.

4. Note, "Medicare's Prospective Payment System: Can Quality Care Survive?" *Iowa Law Review* 69 (1984): 1418.

5. Marmor, *Understanding Health Care Reform,* 51–57.

6. Board of Trustees, "Integration of the Health Care Sector: Definitions, Trends and Implications," in *Proceedings of the House of Delegates* (1985), 105.

7. *Wall Street Journal,* 1 Dec. 1993.

8. Marc A. Rodwin, *Medicine, Money, and Morals: Physicians' Conflicts of Interest* (New York: Oxford University Press, 1993), 16–17.

9. Marmor, *Understanding Health Care Reform,* 32–47.

10. Schattschneider, *Semisovereign People,* 10 (emphasis in original).

11. See, e.g., American Medical Ass'n v. United States, 317 U.S. 519 (1943). This case was an exception to the rule because the indictments of AMA officials for restraint of trade occurred in the District of Columbia where federal jurisdiction was not an issue.

12. U.S. v. Oregon State Medical Society, 343 U.S. 326 (1952); Riggall v. Washington County Medical Society, 249 F.2d 266 (8th Cir. 1957); Speers Free Clinic and Hospital v. Cleere, 197 F.2d 125 (10th Cir. 1952).

13. See Philip C. Kissam, William L. Webber, Lawrence W. Bigus, and John R. Holzgraefe, "Antitrust and Hospital Privileges: Testing the Conventional Wisdom," *California Law Review* 70 (1982): 619.

14. Berlant, *Profession and Monopoly,* 238.

15. DHEW, *Report on Licensure* (1971): 43–52; Walter Gelhorn, "The Abuse of Occupational Licensing," *University of Chicago Law Review* 44 (1976): 6–27; Milton Friedman, *Capitalism and Freedom* (Chicago: University of Chicago Press, 1962).

16. See DHEW, *Developments in Licensure; Credentialing Health Manpower,* 10–11.

17. Kenneth W. Clarkson and Timothy J. Muris, "Constraining the Federal Trade Commission: The Case of Occupational Regulation," *University of Miami Law Review* 35 (1980): 110–12.

18. 317 U.S. 341 (1942).

19. 433 U.S. 350 (1977).

20. In the Matter of American Medical Association, Docket No. 9064. The order forbid AMA action that would "(1) restrict its members' solicitation of patients by advertising, submission of bids, or other means; (2) interfere with either the amount or the form of compensation provided a member in exchange for his or her professional services, in contracts with entities offering physician services to the public; (3) characterize as unethical the use of closed panel or other health care delivery plans that limit the patient's choice of a physician; (4) characterize as unethical the participation of non-physicians in the ownership or management of health care organizations that provide physician services to the public."

21. 421 U.S. 556 (1975).

22. American Medical Association v. Federal Trade Commission, 455 U.S. 676 (1982).

23. Edward B. Hirshfeld, AMA, and John M. Peterson, counsel for Chicago Medical Society, to Donald S. Clark, secretary, Federal Trade Commission, 23 Jan. 1992, Special Collections, AMA.

24. Board of Trustees, "Peer Review after *Patrick v. Burget,*" in *Proceedings of the House of Delegates* (1988), 3–4; Note, "The Health Care Quality Improvement Act of 1986: Will Physicians Find Peer Review More Inviting?" *Virginia Law Review* 74 (1988): 1116–18; Alan M. Rifkin, Gerard E. Evans, and Greg D. Hall, "Antitrust's Recent Attack on the Peer Review Practitioner: Is the Health Care Quality Improvement Act a Viable Remedy?" *Maryland Medical Journal* (Jan. 1990): 22.

25. Kissam, "Antitrust and Hospital Privileges," 599.

26. See Hospital Building Co. v. Trustees of Rex Hospital, 425 U.S. 738 (1976).

27. Board of Trustees, "Peer Review after *Patrick*," 5.

28. Kissam, "Antitrust and Hospital Privileges," 642–48.

29. Ibid., 671.

30. 486 U.S. 94 (1988). Discussions and interpretations of the *Patrick* case appear in numerous medical and legal journals. See, e.g., William J. Curran, "Legal Immunity for Medical Peer-Review Programs," *New England Journal of Medicine* 320 (1989): 233–35.

31. Cf. Mor J. McCarthy, "The Professional Liability Crisis from the Standpoint of Physicians and Hospitals," *Federation Bulletin* 63 (Oct. 1976): 325–39; Barry R. Furrow et al., *Health Law: Cases, Materials and Problems,* 2d ed., American Casebook Series (St. Paul: West Publishing, 1991), 379–89.

32. Joseph I. Pines, "The Need for Medico-Legal Cooperation in Treating Malpractice Suits," *Maryland State Medical Journal* (Jan. 1970): 90–91.

33. Furrow, *Health Law,* 381, 392–95.

34. George S. Palmer, "Effective Discipline of Incompetent Physicians: Number One Problem and Need of State Licensing Boards," *Federation Bulletin* 65 (Apr. 1978): 120; Grad and Marti, *Physician's Licensure and Discipline,* 3–4.

35. Harold E. Wilkins, "California Legislature Establishes Board of Medical Quality Assurance," *Federation Bulletin* 63 (Jan. 1976): 13.

36. William E. Drips Jr., "Physician Discipline in Oregon," *Federation Bulletin* 75 (Sept. 1988): 299.

37. Claude E. Welch, "The New Massachusetts Board of Registration and Discipline in Medicine," *Federation Bulletin* 63 (Sept. 1976): 299–301.

38. 411 U.S. 564 (1973).

39. 440 U.S. 1 (1979).

40. See Cohen, "Professional Power and Conflict of Interest," 10–12, 17–19.

41. The work was published in 1979, but the sample year was 1976. See Grad and Marti, *Physician's Licensure and Discipline,* 413.

42. Actually, the federation began compiling information on board structure and composition in a statistical format in 1986. Not enough boards responded to the federation's request for information on membership status in 1986 to allow comparison for statistical purposes.

43. Howard L. Horns, "Challenges to and Responsibilities of the Federation of State Medical Boards," *Federation Bulletin* 62 (Mar. 1975): 81.

44. Cohen, "Professional Power and Conflict of Interest," 20; William K. Selden, "Licensing Boards Are Archaic," *American Journal of Nursing* 70 (Jan. 1970): 125; Benjamin Shimberg and Doug Roederer, *Occupational Licensing: Questions a Legislator Should Ask* (Lexington, Ky.: Council of State Governments, 1978), 20–21.

45. Grad and Marti, *Physician's Licensure and Discipline,* 115.

46. Dolan and Urban, "Effectiveness of Medical Disciplinary Boards," 216.

47. Grad and Marti, *Physician's Licensure and Discipline*, 57.

48. Derbyshire, *Medical Licensure*, 34, 35.

49. AMA, *Report of the Medical Disciplinary Committee* (1961), 54.

50. Grad and Marti, *Physician's Licensure and Discipline*, App. A.

51. Federation of State Medical Boards, *Exchange* (1986): 6–7; (1995–96): 6–7. It is possible that some state medical boards either failed to respond or provided the federation with incomplete or inaccurate information in 1986, which would account for the small increase in the number of state societies having a designated role in the nominating process in 1996. Minor discrepancies should not detract from my conclusions, which are based on long-term trends.

52. Grad and Marti, *Physician's Licensure and Discipline*, 38.

53. See Federation of State Medical Boards, *Exchange* (1995–96): 38–39.

54. Drips, "Physician Discipline in Oregon," 299.

55. See Annual Reports of the Maryland Board of Physician Quality Assurance for the years 1986 and 1987.

56. Henry S. Patterson II, *Report and Recommendations of the State of New Jersey Commission of Investigation on Impaired and Incompetent Physicians* (Trenton: New Jersey State Commission on Investigation, 1987), 37 (hereafter SCI Report).

57. James S. Todd, "Identifying Problem Physicians: Channels of Information," *Federation Bulletin* 74 (Jan. 1987): 5–6. See also John H. Morton, "Controlling Medical Incompetence," *Federation Bulletin* 62 (Aug. 1975): 275.

58. Richard P. Kusserow, "The State Boards: Perceptions of the OIG," *Federation Bulletin* 74 (Nov. 1987): 328–29.

59. Gross, *Of Foxes and Hen Houses*, 111.

60. *Washington Post*, 1 Sept. 1985; *New York Times*, 2 Sept. 1985.

61. Elton Rayack, "Medical Licensure: Social Costs and Social Benefits," *Law and Human Behavior* 7, nos. 2/3 (1983): 154–55; Daniel B. Hogan, "The Effectiveness of Licensing: History, Evidence, and Recommendations," *Law and Human Behavior* 7, nos. 2/3 (1983): 124–25; Gelhorn, "Abuse of Occupational Licensing," 16–17; Gross, *Of Foxes and Hen Houses*, 147–51.

62. Gross, *Of Foxes and Hen Houses*, 94–97; Grad and Marti, *Physician's Licensure and Discipline*, 234, n. 229.

63. Gregory W. Schroeder, "Board Reorganization, Umbrella Agencies, Super Boards: Pro's and Con's," *Federation Bulletin* 68 (Oct. 1981): 300; Gross, *Of Foxes and Hen Houses*, 94.

64. Derbyshire, *Medical Licensure*, xi–xii; Bernard J. Pisani, "Assuring Continuing Professional Competence," *Federation Bulletin* 63 (Sept. 1976): 259; Schroeder, "Board Reorganization," 291.

65. DHHS, OIG, *Medical Licensure and Discipline; State Medical Boards and Medical Discipline* (Boston: Office of Evaluations and Inspections, 1990).

66. Congress, House, Committee on Ways and Means, and Committee on Energy and the Environment, *Medicare and Medicaid Patient Protection Act of 1984*, 98th Cong., 2d session, 1984; Congress, House, Committee on Energy and Com-

merce, *The Health Care Quality Improvement Act of 1986: Hearing before the Subcommittee on Health and the Environment,* 99th Cong., 2d session, 18 Mar. 1986; Congress, House, Committee on Small Business, *Can State Boards Protect the Public? Hearing before the Subcommittee on Regulation, Business Opportunities, and Energy,* 101 Cong., 2d session, 8 June (1990).

67. The Hippocratic Oath and Percival's Code are forerunners of the modern version adopted by the AMA. AMA, *Code of Medical Ethics,* ix–x.

68. Robert M. Tenery, "County, State Medical Societies Shouldn't Be Forgotten," *American Medical News,* 7 Aug. 1995, 14.

69. See Cindy Anne Stearns, "Company Doctors: A Study of HMO Control over Medical Work" (Ph.D. dissertation, University of California, Davis, 1988), 264–66.

70. Marc L. Rivo and David Satcher, "Improving Access to Health Care through Physician Workforce Reform," *JAMA* 270 (Sept. 1, 1993): 1076.

71. Congressional hearings on the Health Care Quality Improvement Act of 1986 (testimony of Willis B. Goldbeck, president, Washington Business Group on Health), 379.

72. By way of example, forty-two hospitals closed in 1993. This was consistent with trends reported for 1987–92. DHHS, OIG, "Hospital Closures: 1993."

73. Starr, *Social Transformation,* 428–29.

74. Cf. Emanuel and Emanuel, "Preserving Community in Health Care," 157.

75. Marie R. Haug, "Deprofessionalization: An Alternative Hypothesis for the Future," *Sociological Review Monographs* 20 (1973): 195–211; "A Re-examination of the Hypothesis of Physician Deprofessionalization," *Millbank Quarterly* 66, supp. 2 (1988): 48–56.

76. Samuel P. Hays, "The Politics of Environmental Administration," in *The New American State: Bureaucracies and Policies since World War II,* ed. Louis Galambos (Baltimore: Johns Hopkins University Press, 1987), 23.

77. Mark R. Yessian, "From Self-regulation to Public Protection: Medical Licensure Authorities in an Age of Rising Consumerism," *Federation Bulletin* 81, no. 3 (1994): 190–94.

78. Schattschneider, *Semisovereign People,* 11.

Chapter 3. Building a Modern State Medical Board

1. See Richard H. Hall, "Professionalisation and Bureaucratisation," in *People and Organizations,* ed. Graeme Salaman and Kenneth Thompson (London: Open University, 1973), 120–25.

2. DHHS, OIG Report, *State Medical Boards and Medical Discipline,* 8.

3. Grad and Marti, *Physician's Licensure and Discipline,* 22; Schroeder, "Board Reorganization," 298–99; congressional hearings on physician discipline (1990) (comments of Representative Ron Wyden), 1–2.

4. Cf. AMA, *Report of the Medical Disciplinary Committee,* 52; Derbyshire, "Medical Self-regulation," 198.

5. Wylie, "Doctors' Conspiracy of Silence," 180.

6. AMA, *Report of the Medical Disciplinary Committee* (1961), 31; James Winn, M.D., executive vice president, Federation of State Medical Boards, interview by author, 21 Mar. 1995.

7. Minutes of the Board of Medical Examiners of the State of Maryland from 1955 to 1969, Special Collections, Maryland Board of Physician Quality Assurance. Interview by author of James Winn, M.D., 21 Mar. 1995.

8. Kenneth C. Yohn, "FSMB—Protection of the Public a Primary Function," *Federation Bulletin* 75 (Aug. 1988): 240; Dale G. Breaden, "Concentrating on the Problem Physician: Perspectives in Medical Discipline—Part II," *Federation Bulletin* 76 (Mar. 1989): 78.

9. Philip K. Howard, *The Death of Common Sense: How Law Is Suffocating America* (New York: Random House, 1994), 81.

10. 353 U.S. 232 (1957).

11. Grad and Marti, *Physician's Licensure and Discipline,* 141–59; AMA Law Division, *Disciplinary Digest,* 34–58.

12. Charles L. Terry Jr., "Physician as Defendant," 26.

13. In a significant ruling for disciplinary bodies, the U.S. Supreme Court held that combining investigatory, prosecutorial, and adjudicative functions in a single agency did not per se violate due process. Withrow v. Larkin, 421 U.S. 35 (1975).

14. Before the 1970s, medical practice acts in most states limited the range of sanctions to probation, suspension, or revocation of a physician's license. Boards were reluctant to impose these severe penalties in most cases. Grad and Marti, *Physician's Licensure and Discipline,* 42, 173–77; Robert A. Chase, "What to Do about the Incompetent Physician?" *Federation Bulletin* 64 (June 1977): 172. Since the 1970s, the trend has been toward more flexible sanctions. Boards in the 1990s have the power to issue fines and reprimands or enter into consent agreements that permit physicians to continue practicing while undergoing rehabilitation. See Federation of State Medical Boards, *Exchange* (1995–96), 54–55.

15. Even after the revocation of a physician's license, courts in several states could stay the board's order pending judicial review. Derbyshire, "Medical Self-regulation," 199. Courts in many states are no longer permitted to do this. See, e.g., Maryland Medical Practice Act (1993), sec. 14-408(c).

16. The standard in most instances was "clear and convincing evidence" that exceeds the "preponderance of evidence" standard in civil cases. See DHHS, OIG Report, *State Medical Boards and Medical Discipline* (1990), 9. Twenty-two state medical boards retain the "clear and convincing evidence" standard. Foundation of State Medical Boards, *Exchange* (1995–96), 72.

17. Many states had administrative procedure acts that prohibited communications between the trier of fact and parties to adjudicatory proceedings. Grad and Marti, *Physician's Licensure and Discipline,* 143, 153–54.

18. I experienced this on many occasions as legal counsel to Maryland's Com-

mission on Medical Discipline, predecessor to the Maryland Board of Physician Quality Assurance.

19. Grad and Marti, *Physician's Licensure and Discipline,* 146.

20. Federation of State Medical Boards, *Exchange* (1986): 28.

21. Wolfe et al., *Questionable Doctors* (1996), 1.

22. Grad and Marti, *Physician's Licensure and Discipline,* 164–68.

23. See, e.g., *Minneapolis Star and Tribune Co. v. Minnesota State Board of Medical Examiners,* 282 Minn. 86, 165 N.W. 2d 46 (1968).

24. Federation of State Medical Boards, *Exchange* (1995–96): 58–59.

25. Anne Paxton, "The Tide against Secrecy," *Federation Bulletin* 80 (winter 1993): 236.

26. DHHS, OIG Report, *Medical Licensure and Discipline,* 16.

27. Cf. Bernard J. Pisani, "Assuring Continuing Professional Competence," *Federation Bulletin* 63 (Sept. 1976): 259.

28. The Health Care Quality Improvement Act of 1986, Pub. L. No. 99-660, secs. 401–32, 100 Stat. 3784 (1986) (codified at 42 U.S.C.A. secs. 11), 101–11, 152 (West Supp. 1988), *amended by* Pub. L. No. 100-77, sec. 402, 101 Stat. 986, 1007 (1987) (codified at U.S.C. sec. 11,137).

29. Congressional hearings on the Health Care Quality Improvement Act of 1986 (comments of Representative Henry Waxman), 191; John K. Iglehart, "Congress Moves to Bolster Peer Review: The Health Care Quality Improvement Act of 1986," *New England Journal of Medicine* 316 (1987): 963; Henry A. Waxman, "Medical Malpractice and Quality of Care," *New England Journal of Medicine* 316 (1987): 943–44.

30. Breaden, "Concentrating on the Problem Physician—Part II," 78, 81.

31. C. John Tupper, "Bad Apples Versus Good Eggs: A Look at Quality, Professionalism and Health Access America," *Federation Bulletin* 78 (Sept. 1991): 262.

32. Norbert W. Budde, "Data Bank Operation: A Perspective," *Federation Bulletin* 76 (Apr. 1989): 103.

33. Tupper, "Bad Apples," 263 (emphasis in original).

34. See VanTuinen et al., *Questionable Doctors* (1991), 3.

35. See Paxton, "Tide against Secrecy," 236–39; Fleming, "Massachusetts Physician Profiles," 9.

36. Eliot Freidson, "The Medical Profession in Transition," in *Applications of Social Science to Clinical Medicine and Health Policy,* ed. Linda Aiken and David Mechanic (New Brunswick, N.J.: Rutgers University Press, 1986), 214.

37. Ibid., 223.

38. Kusserow et al., "Overview of State Medical Discipline," 822.

39. *A Guide to the Essentials of a Modern Medical Practice Act,* 6 (emphasis in original).

40. Schroeder, "Board Reorganization," 291, 301.

41. Cohen, "Professional Power and Conflict of Interest," 21, n. 36.

42. U.S. Department of Labor, *Occupational Licensing and the Supply of Non-*

professional Manpower, Manpower Research Monograph no. 11 (Washington, D.C.: U.S. Government Printing Office, 1969), 3.

43. Cohen, "Professional Power and Conflict of Interest," 21.

44. Taskforce on Health Care Workforce Regulation, *Reforming Health Care Workforce Regulation: Policy Considerations for the 21st Century* (San Francisco: Pew Health Professions Commission, 1995), 14.

45. Ibid., 16.

46. Editorial, "The Legislator Examines Malpractice," *Federation Bulletin* 62 (Aug. 1975): 252.

47. Grad and Marti, *Physician's Licensure and Discipline,* 234, n. 229.

48. Joseph A. Riggs, "Regulations, Licensure, Medical Discipline, and Self-regulation of Physicians," *Journal of the Medical Society of New Jersey* 76 (Feb. 1979): 109–11; Gross, *Foxes and Hen Houses,* 94.

49. Gross, *Foxes and Hen Houses,* 94.

50. DHHS, OIG Report, *Medical Licensure and Discipline: An Overview* (1986), 12, 16.

51. Congressional hearings on physician discipline (1990) (testimony of John Ulwelling, executive director, Oregon State Board of Medical Examiners), 36.

52. Grad and Marti, *Physician's Licensure and Discipline,* 422–26; congressional hearings on physician discipline (1990) (testimony of Laura Wittkin, executive director, Stop Hospital and Medical Error), 5–6.

53. DHHS, OIG Report, *State Medical Boards and Medical Discipline,* 8.

54. Congressional hearings on physician discipline (1990) (testimony of Laura Wittkin), 6.

55. Freidson, "Medical Profession in Transition," 63–79.

56. Eliot Freidson, "The Reorganization of the Medical Profession," *Medical Care Review* 42 (spring 1985): 24–33; "The Changing Nature of Professional Control," *Annual Review of Sociology* 10 (1984): 16–19.

57. Federation of State Medical Boards, *Federation Handbook* (1993).

58. Dale G. Breaden, "Concentrating on the Problem Physician: Perspectives in Medical Discipline—Part I," *Federation Bulletin* 76 (Feb. 1989): 45.

59. The federation promoted the concept of an independent board through its *Guide to the Essentials of a Modern Medical Practice Act,* first published in 1956 and revised in 1970, 1977, 1985, 1988, 1991, and 1994.

60. David A. Citron, *Guide to the Essentials of a Modern Medical Practice Act* (Fort Worth, Tex.: Federation of State Medical Boards, 1988), 4–5.

61. Andrew and Sauer, "Do Boards of Medicine Really Matter?" 234.

62. Citron, *Guide to the Essentials of a Modern Medical Practice Act,* 4.

63. Sigel, *Elements of a Modern State Medical Board,* 1–13.

64. Federally sponsored peer review organizations (PROs) used professional associations to monitor the necessity and quality of physician services in hospitals on behalf of the federal Medicare program. According to Richard Scott, "PROs represented a compromise between the dominant structural interests of the profes-

sional monopolists and the challenging structural interests of the corporate rationalizers." Scott, "Health Care Organizations in the 1980s," 110. Compromise or not, organized medicine strongly resented the intrusion of the federal government on its professional turf and, for many years, favored substantial modifications to the PRO program. See, e.g., Board of Trustees, "PRO Legislation Repeal," in *Proceedings of the House of Delegates* (1987), 69–70.

65. Schattschneider, *Semisovereign People,* 41.

66. *Guide to the Essentials of a Modern Medical Practice Act,* 31.

67. Quinn, "What We're Doing about the Bad Apples," 232, 234.

68. McKeown, "Present Status of Medical Discipline," 140; Grad and Marti, *Physician's Licensure and Discipline,* 119–20.

69. Federation of State Medical Boards, *Exchange* (1986): 18; (1995–96): 21.

70. Ibid. (1995–96): 2–3.

71. Since the passage of legislation in 1991, New York's Board of Professional Medical Conduct, which is in the Department of Health, has final decision-making authority. Although the federation designates the board "advisory," it is currently "semi-autonomous." Ansell Marks, Executive Secretary, Board of Professional Medical Conduct, telephone interview by author, 31 July 1997.

72. Federation of State Medical Boards, *Exchange* (1986): 16.

73. Ibid. (1992–93): 50–51.

74. Andrew and Sauer, "Do Boards of Medicine Really Matter?" 234.

Chapter 4. Balancing Public and Professional Concerns

1. The federation does not include in its official summaries a breakdown of the reasons for disciplinary actions. Consequently, the data contained in figure 4.1 come from unofficial sources. Derbyshire compiled the data for the years 1963 to 1967. Public Citizen compiled the data for the years 1986 to 1996. Public Citizen issued the following disclaimer in the 1996 edition of *Questionable Doctors*: "Please note that the period of years covered in our database varies from state to state—e.g., we may have received disciplinary materials covering six years for one state but only three years for another state. Therefore, our statistics should not be viewed as nationally representative for any specific time period." Wolfe et al., *Questionable Doctors* (1996), 17. Despite these problems in data collection and compilation, the information is useful for showing certain long-term trends. Reliable data concerning types of case dispositions for the period 1967–86 are unavailable.

2. For drug and alcohol abuse, see Council on Mental Health, "The Sick Physician: Impairment by Psychiatric Disorders, Including Alcoholism and Drug Dependence," *JAMA* 223 (Feb. 5, 1973): 684–87; Barbara S. Schneidman, "Report of the Ad Hoc Committee on Physician Impairment," *Federation Bulletin* 81, no. 4 (1994): 229–42. For sexual misconduct, see Council on Ethical and Judicial Affairs, "Sexual Misconduct in the Practice of Medicine," *JAMA* 266 (20 Nov. 1991): 2741–45; Barbara S. Schneidman, *Report on Sexual Boundary Issues from the Ad Hoc Committee on Physician Impairment* (Euless, Tex.: Federation of State Medical Boards,

1995). For incompetence, see Council on Medical Service, "Principles for Voluntary Medical Peer Review: An Interim Report," in *Proceedings of the House of Delegates* (1981); Porter, "Ethics and Quality of Care."

3. Randolph P. Reaves, "Sexual Intimacies with Patients: The Regulatory Issue of the Nineties," *Federation Bulletin* 80, no. 2 (1993): 83–89.

4. See, e.g., "Maryland Moves to Punish Bad Doctors: Bill Would Toughen Physician Discipline," *Washington Post,* 7 Apr. 1988; "Panel OKs Therapist Regulation; State Bills Would Criminalize Sexual Contact with Patients," *Boston Globe,* 24 Jan. 1990.

5. See, e.g., "Psychotherapy: Doctors Sleeping with Patients—A Growing Crisis of Ethical Abuse," *Newsweek,* 13 Apr. 1992; "Doctors Rarely Lose Licenses; Maryland Panel Allowed Rapist to Keep Practicing," *Washington Post,* 10 Jan. 1988; "Panel Likely to Clear Doctor of Sex Abuse; Critics Decry Handling of Women's Complaints," *Boston Globe,* 3 July 1992; Sabrina Rubin, "Intimate Intimidation," *Philadelphia* (Apr. 1996): 108–16.

6. DHHS, OIG, *State Medical Boards and Quality of Care Cases: Promising Approaches* (Boston: Office of Evaluation and Inspections, 1993), 4–24.

7. *Washington Post,* 10, 11 Jan. 1988.

8. Stanley R. Platman and Michael C. Llufrio, "The Physician Rehabilitation Program of Maryland," *Maryland Medical Journal* (Nov. 1990): 1029; Council on Mental Health, "The Sick Physician," 684.

9. Platman and Llufrio, "Physician Rehabilitation Program," 1029; William T. Dixon, "The Case of the Emotionally-Ill Doctor: Physician, Heal Thyself," *Maryland State Medical Journal* (Oct. 1980): 55.

10. Gerald L. Summer, "Physician Impairment: Current Concepts," *Federation Bulletin* 81, no. 2 (1994): 121.

11. Jerome E. Coller, "The Maryland Physician Rehabilitation Committee Program," *Maryland State Medical Journal* (Oct. 1980): 36; Kathryn L. Sprinkle, "Physicians Alcoholism: A Survey of the Literature," *Federation Bulletin* 81, no. 2 (1994): 113–19.

12. Derbyshire, *Medical Licensure,* 80.

13. Council on Mental Health, "The Sick Physician," 686.

14. Grad and Marti, *Physician's Licensure and Discipline,* 159–63.

15. Derbyshire, "Medical Self-regulation," 200.

16. Grad and Marti, *Physician's Licensure and Discipline,* 161.

17. Linda C. Chandler, "The Philosophy of Rehabilitation for Impaired Physicians," *Federation Bulletin* 82, no. 3 (1995): 125.

18. S. Lon Conner, "Comparison of Impaired Physicians Programs Nationwide," *Maryland Medical Journal* 37 (Mar. 1988): 214; Robert Kane White and Edward J. Kitlowski, "Physicians in Recovery," *Maryland Medical Journal* 37 (Mar. 1988): 189.

19. See, e.g., Council on Ethical and Judicial Affairs, "Reporting Impaired,

Incompetent, or Unethical Colleagues," in *Reports of the Council on Ethical and Judicial Affairs of the AMA* (Chicago: American Medical Association, 1991), 28.

20. Council on Mental Health, "The Sick Physician," 684–87.

21. Robert Kane White and Michael Gilbert Hayes, "The Physician Rehabilitation Program of Maryland," *Maryland Medical Journal* 36 (Mar. 1987): 221.

22. The vast majority of IPPs are physician sponsored. In some states, boards have their own IPPs or operate them under a joint arrangement with the state medical society. See Federation of State Medical Boards, *Exchange* (1992–93): 69. When referring to IPPs, I mean physician-sponsored programs.

23. Platman and Llufrio, "Physician Rehabilitation Program," 1005.

24. Robert C. Vanderberry, "The North Carolina Physicians Health Program," *Federation Bulletin* 82, no. 3 (1995): 146.

25. See, e.g., White and Hayes, "Physician Rehabilitation Program of Maryland," 221; Frederick Alpern et al., "A Survey of Recovering Maryland Physicians," *Maryland Medical Journal* (Apr. 1992): 301–3; Edward G. Reading, "Nine Years Experience with Chemically Dependent Physicians: The New Jersey Experience," *Maryland Medical Journal* (Apr. 1992): 325–29.

26. Chandler, "Philosophy of Rehabilitation," 125.

27. White and Kitlowski, "Physicians in Recovery," 189; Edward T. Carden, "Whither the Impaired Physician? The Politics of Impairment," *Maryland Medical Journal* (Mar. 1988): 206.

28. White and Hayes, "Physician Rehabilitation Program of Maryland," 221 (Maryland experience); Reading, "Nine Years," 327–28 (New Jersey experience).

29. Carden, "Wither the Impaired Physician," 210, 206.

30. G. Douglas Talbott, "The Impaired Physician Movement," *Maryland Medical Journal* (Mar. 1988): 216.

31. See Donna M. Dorsey and Roslyn Scheer, "Licensing Boards and Impaired Professionals," *Maryland Medical Journal* (Mar. 1987): 238. Dorsey, executive director for Maryland's board of nursing, and Scheer, executive director for Maryland's board of pharmacy, relate the general experience among board administrators in the 1980s. The federation's 1988 survey reflects the prevalence of IPPs and their growing relationship with boards in several states. Federation of State Medical Boards, *Exchange* (1988): 51–52.

32. Talbott, "Impaired Physician Movement," 216.

33. SCI Report, 13.

34. Jeffrey Kanige, "SCI Fighting for Its Life," *New Jersey Law Journal* (3 Jan. 1994): 56.

35. SCI Report, 20.

36. Ibid., 8, 10.

37. Ibid., 18, 74.

38. Clark Martin, "Governmental Affairs Update," *New Jersey Medicine* 85 (Mar. 1988): 84.

39. Carden, "Wither the Impaired Physician," 206.

40. N.J. Stat. Ann., sec. 26:2H-12.2 (West Supp. 1989).

41. Sean Patrick Murphy, "Professional Medical Conduct Reform Act," *New Jersey Medicine* 87 (Dec. 1990): 991.

42. See Medical Society of New Jersey v. Jacobs, Civil No. 93-3670, slip op. at 3–4 (D.N.J. Oct. 5, 1993).

43. Linda Oberman, "Sensitive Licensure Questions Criticized: Judge, Justice Dept. Back N.J. Doctors' Suit," *American Medical News,* 25 Oct. 1993, 1, 37.

44. Hirsch v. New Jersey State Board of Medical Examiners, 128 N.J. 160 (1992), aff'g, 252 N.J. Super 596 (App. Div. 1991).

45. Memorandum of the United States as *amicus curiae, Jacobs,* 3, 14, 19, 20, n. 24.

46. *Jacobs,* 14.

47. Katherine M. Carroll, executive director, Medical Practitioner Review Panel, Board of Medical Examiners of New Jersey, telephone interview by author, 31 Jan. 1996.

48. Relicensure Application of the Board of Physician Quality Assurance of the State of Maryland, 1993. See also Oberman, "Sensitive Licensure Questions," 37.

49. Vanderberry, "North Carolina Physicians Health Program," 146.

50. See Paxton, "Tide against Secrecy," 236.

51. Public Health Service Act, secs. 527 and 523, 42 U.S.C. 290ee-3 and 290dd-3. For state medical records acts, see, e.g., Md. Code Ann., *Health-General,* secs. 4-301–9.

52. 42 C.F.R., sec. 2.13.

53. Shoemaker v. Handel, 608 F.Supp. 1151 (D.C.N.J. 1985); Dr. K v. State Board, 632 A.2d 453 (Md. App. 1993).

54. State Board of Medical Examiners v. Fenwick Hall Inc., No. 23672 (S.C. Sup. Ct. June 8, 1992).

55. SCI Report, 8; David I. Canavan, "Confrontation," *Journal of the Medical Society of New Jersey* 80 (May 1983): 369–70.

56. Carden, "Wither the Impaired Physician," 208.

57. Ibid., 207.

58. Roger A. Goetz, "The Florida Impaired Practitioners Program," Burns M. Brady, "Kentucky Physicians Health Foundation Impaired Physicians Program," and Lynn Hankes, "Washington Physicians Health Program," in *Federal Bulletin* 82, no. 3 (1995): 131, 137, 158. See also Vanderberry, "North Carolina Physicians Health Program," 147.

59. See Penelope P. Ziegler, "The Physicians' Health Programs of the Educational and Scientific Trust of the Pennsylvania Medical Society" *Federation Bulletin* 82, no. 3 (1995): 152.

60. Schneidman, *Report of Committee on Physician Impairment,* 3.

61. Professional Assistance Program Approval Agreement, 14 June 1995.

62. Council on Ethical and Judicial Affairs, "Sexual Misconduct," 2741.

63. Ibid. See also Ludwig Edelstein, *The Hippocratic Oath: Text, Translation and Interpretation* (Baltimore: Johns Hopkins Press, 1943), 3.

64. Council on Ethical and Judicial Affairs, "Sexual Misconduct," 2742.

65. Larry H. Strasburger, Linda Jorgenson, and Paul Sutherland, "The Prevention of Psychotherapist Sexual Misconduct: Avoiding the Slippery Slope," *American Journal of Psychotherapy* 46, no. 4 (1992): 545.

66. Linda Jorgenson and Rebecca Randles, "Time Out: The Statute of Limitations and Fiduciary Theory in Psychotherapist Sexual Misconduct Cases," *Oklahoma Law Review* 44, no. 2 (1991): 196–203.

67. Roy v. Hartogs, 81 Misc.2d 350, 352, 366 N.Y.S.2d 297, 299 (N.Y. Civ. Ct. 1975); Horak v. Biris, 474 N.E.2d 13 (Ill. 1985).

68. Council on Ethical and Judicial Affairs, "Sexual Misconduct," 2741.

69. Nanette K. Gartrell et al., "Psychotherapist-Patient Sexual Contact: Results of a National Survey. I: Prevalence," *American Journal of Psychiatry* 143 (1986): 1126–31.

70. Nanette K. Gartrell et al., "Reporting Practices of Psychiatrists Who Knew of Sexual Misconduct by Colleagues," *American Journal of Orthopsychiatry* 57 (1987): 287–95.

71. Council on Ethical and Judicial Affairs, "Sexual Misconduct," 2741.

72. Nanette K. Gartrell et al., "Physician-Patient Sexual Contact: Prevalence and Problems," *Western Journal of Medicine* 157 (1992): 140–43.

73. Glen O. Gabbard, "Sexual Misconduct," in *Review of Psychiatry,* ed. John M. Oldham and Michelle B. Riba (Washington, D.C.: American Psychiatry Press, 1994), 436.

74. Council on Ethical and Judicial Affairs, "Sexual Misconduct," 2741.

75. Schneidman, *Report on Sexual Boundary Issues,* 1–2.

76. Council on Ethical and Judicial Affairs, "Sexual Misconduct," 2741.

77. Strasburger, "Prevention of Sexual Misconduct," 546–48.

78. Shirley Feldman-Summers, "Sexual Contact in Fiduciary Relationships," in *Sexual Exploitation in Professional Relationships,* ed. Glen O. Gabbard (Washington, D.C.: American Psychiatric Press, 1989), 201–5.

79. Simmons v. United States, 805 F.2d 1363, 1365–66 (9th Cir. 1986). The court in *Simmons* cites ten cases for this proposition.

80. Linda Jorgenson, Rebecca Randles, and Larry Strasburger, "The Furor over Psychotherapist-Patient Sexual Contact: New Solutions to an Old Problem," *William and Mary Law Review* 32 (spring 1991): 649.

81. Gabbard, "Sexual Misconduct," 433.

82. James R. Winn, "Medical Boards and Sexual Misconduct: An Overview of Federation Data," *Federation Bulletin* 80, no. 2 (1993): 92.

83. Reaves, "Sexual Intimacies with Patients," 84–85.

84. Gabbard, "Sexual Misconduct," 446; Jorgenson et al., "Furor over Psychotherapist-Patient Sexual Contact," 662.

85. Feldman-Summers, "Sexual Contact in Fiduciary Relations," 205.

86. Gabbard, "Sexual Misconduct," 446.

87. Kenneth S. Pope, "How Clients Are Harmed by Sexual Contact with Mental Health Professionals: The Syndrome and Its Prevalence," *Journal of Counseling and Development* 67 (Dec. 1988): 224.

88. Gabbard, "Sexual Misconduct," 437–38.

89. Council on Psychiatry and Law, *Resource Document: Legal Sanctions for Mental Health Professional-Patient Sex* (Washington, D.C.: American Psychiatric Association, 1993).

90. Robert S. Walzer and Stephen Miltimore, "Proctoring of Disciplined Health Care Professionals: Implementation and Model Regulations," *Federation Bulletin* 81, no. 2 (1994): 88–89; Shirley Moskow, "Seeking Strategies against the Stresses of Medicine," *American Medical News,* 1 Jan. 1996, 6.

91. Council on Ethical and Judicial Affairs, "Sexual Misconduct," 2742.

92. Gabbard, "Sexual Misconduct," 440–41; Counsel on Psychiatry and Law, *Resource Document,* 6.

93. See Independent Task Force on Sexual Abuse of Patients, *The Final Report* (Toronto, Ontario: College of Physicians and Surgeons of Ontario, 1991), 104.

94. Gary Richard Schoener, "Employer/Supervisor Liability and Risk Management: An Administrator's View," in *The Breach of Trust: Sexual Exploitation by Health Care Professionals and Clergy,* ed. John Gonsiorek (Thousand Oaks, Calif.: Sage Publications, 1995), 304.

95. See Maryland Board of Physician Quality Assurance, "More on the Use of Chaperones," *BPQA Newsletter* 3 (June 1995): 3.

96. Gross, *Foxes and Hen Houses,* 41–44.

97. Simmons v. United States, 805 F.2d at 1364–65; Gromis v. Medical Board of California, 8 Cal. App. 4th 589, 10 Cal. Rptr. 452 (1992); St. Paul Fire & Marine v. Love, 459 N.W.2d 698 (Minn. 1990).

98. Linda Jorgenson, presentation before the Maryland Task Force on Health Professional–Client Sexual Exploitation, 25 May 1994.

99. Wolfe et al., *Questionable Doctors* (1993), 16.

100. Ralph A. Deterling, *Annual Report to the General Court and the Special Commission on Medical Malpractice* (Boston: Board of Registration in Medicine, 1987), 1.

101. Andrew G. Bodnar, *Annual Report to the General Court and the Special Commission on Medical Malpractice* (Boston: Board of Registration in Medicine, 1988), 37.

102. Deterling, *Annual Report,* 2.

103. Ibid., 1, 3.

104. Paul G. Gitlin, *Annual Report to the General Court and the Special Commission on Medical Malpractice* (Boston: Board of Registration in Medicine, 1990–93), 2.

105. Paul R. McGinn, "Mass. MDs Support Defense of Sanctioned Physician," *American Medical News,* 1 Sept. 1989, 1, 6.

106. Gitlin, *Annual Report*, 2.

107. Larry H. Strasburger, Linda Jorgenson, and Rebecca Randles, "Criminalization of Psychotherapist-Patient Sex," *American Journal of Psychiatry* 148 (July 1991): 859–63.

108. Linda Jorgenson, presentation before the Maryland Task Force on Health Professional–Client Sexual Exploitation, 25 May 1994.

109. See Walzer and Miltimore, "Proclivity of Health Care Professionals," 88–89. But cf. Cheryl E. Winchell, "Commentary: Sexual Abuse of Patients: Ontario's 'Zero Tolerance' Statute," *Federation Bulletin* 82, no. 1 (1995): 37–39.

110. Starr, *Social Transformation*, 12.

111. Freidson, *Profession of Medicine*, 137.

112. See Board of Trustees, "The Role of the Medical Staff in Hospital Quality Assurance Initiatives," in *Proceedings of the House of Delegates* (1992), 53; James Morone and Gary Belkin, "The Science Illusion and the Triumph of Medical Capitalism," paper delivered at the annual meeting of the American Political Science Association, Chicago, 1995, 1–19.

113. Wolfe, *Medical Malpractice*; congressional hearings on the Health Care Quality Improvement Act of 1986, 2; Deterling, *Annual Report*, 1.

114. *New York Times*, 2 Feb. 1986; Wolfe, *Medical Malpractice*, 2.

115. See Council on Medical Service, "Principles for Voluntary Medical Peer Review," 136; Guo Baogang, "Politics of Medical Peer Review" (Ph.D. dissertation, Brandeis University, 1994), 98–102.

116. Baogang, "Politics of Peer Review," 152.

117. Linda Oberman Prager, "Undoing Case Review: New PRO Contract Will Ax Random Samples, Boost Collaboration with Providers," *American Medical News*, 26 June 1995, 1, 22–23.

118. Mark R. Yessian, "How Can State Medical Boards Compete in the Quality Assurance Marketplace?" *Federation Bulletin* 81, no. 2 (1994): 104.

119. Ibid., 103–4; Council on Medical Service, "Guidelines for Quality Assurance," in *Proceedings of the House of Delegates* (1987), 201; David I. Kingsley and Alexander E. Rodi Sr., "Federal PRO Program Undergoing Fundamental Transformation," *New Jersey Medicine* 89 (May 1992): 401–2.

120. Yessian, "How Can State Medical Boards Compete," 102–4; Linda O. Prager, "Inspector General: Can PROs Effectively Teach and Police?" *American Medical News*, 4 Mar. 1996, 3, 30. See also Geoffrey R. Norman et al., "Competency Assessment of Primary Care Physicians as Part of a Peer Review Program," *JAMA* 270 (Sept. 1, 1993): 1046–51.

121. Congressional hearings on the Health Care Quality Improvement Act of 1986 (statement of the AMA), 442.

122. Paul C. Weiler, *Medical Malpractice on Trial* (Cambridge, Mass.: Harvard University Press, 1991), 79, 129.

123. Iglehart, "Congress Moves to Bolster Peer Review," 960.

124. Maryland Medical Practice Act (1986), ch. 642, sec. 3.

125. Grad and Marti, *Physician's Licensure and Discipline,* 125.

126. See Robert L. Roth, "Analysis of an Incompetence Case," *Maryland Medical Journal* 38 (Jan. 1989): 49–51.

127. Yessian, "State Medical Boards and Quality Assurance," 126–28.

128. DHHS, OIG Report, *State Medical Boards and Quality of Care Cases,* 1.

129. SCI Report, 32–41.

130. See VanTuinen et al., *Questionable Doctors;* Wolfe et al., *Questionable Doctors* (1993); "Panel Has Difficulty Determining Incompetence," *Washington Post,* 11 Jan. 1988; "Tougher Peer Review of Doctors Urged," *New York Times,* 18 June 1985; "Doctors Who Get Away with Killing and Maiming Must Be Stopped," *New York Times,* 2 Feb. 1986; "Who Is Minding the Doctors?" *USA Today,* 29 June 1990; "Deadly Doctors," *Woman's Day,* 12 Oct. 1993; "Is Your Doctor Safe?" *Self,* Nov. 1991.

131. See Yessian, "How Can State Medical Boards Compete," 103–4.

132. Wolfe, *Medical Malpractice;* interview by author of James Winn, 21 Mar. 1995.

133. Arthur Owens, "Peer Review: Is Testifying Worth the Hassle?" *Medical Economics,* 20 Aug. 1984.

134. Council on Medical Service, "Principles for Voluntary Medical Peer Review," 136–40.

135. Cf. Berlant, *Profession and Monopoly,* 240–47.

136. See "Panel Discussion on Peer Review," moderated by Arthur E. Cocco, chairman, Peer Review Committee, in *Maryland State Medical Journal* (Jan. 1973): 42.

137. Philip Whittlesey to Philip Wagley, 26 Feb. 1971, Special Collections, Baltimore City Medical Society.

138. Newsletter of Peer Review Committee, June 1974, Special Collections, Baltimore City Medical Society. See also Report of Peer Review Committee, 1973, Special Collections, Baltimore City Medical Society.

139. Report of Peer Review Committee of Med Chi, Emidio Bianco, chairman, Special Collections, Baltimore City Medical Society.

140. John DeHoff to Emidio Bianco, 18 Mar. 1974, Special Collections, Baltimore City Medical Society.

141. Maryland Medical Practice Act (1968), ch. 469, sec. 145.

142. Alan O'Neill to Donald Pillsbury, 18 Jan. 1978, Special Collections, Library of the Medical and Chirurgical Faculty.

143. David McHold and Constance Townsend, "The Changing Demands of Peer Review: Introduction to the Peer Review Handbook," *Maryland State Medical Journal* (June 1981): 67.

144. Report of the Commission on Medical Discipline, 17 Dec. 1974; Jerome Coller to John Sargeant, 26 Dec. 1974, Special Collections, Baltimore City Medical Society.

145. David McHold to presidents of Component Societies and Chairmen of

Component Society Peer Review Committees, 16 Apr. 1980, Special Collections, Baltimore City Medical Society.

146. Angelo J. Triosi and Gerard E. Evans, "Physician Discipline: A Continuing Challenge," *Maryland Medical Journal* 37 (Sept. 1988): 709–10.

147. Maryland Medical Practice Act (1988), ch. 109, secs. 1–6.

148. "Report Criticizes Maryland's Regulation of Its Doctors," *Baltimore Sun,* 29 June 1990; "State Should Study Oversight of Physicians," *Annapolis Capital,* 1 July 1990; "Medical Board Flaws Persist, Records Show," *Evening Sun,* 1 Mar. 1991; "Doctor Discipline in Maryland Still Found Wanting," *Baltimore Sun,* 17 May 1991; "Review Board Too Tight with Doctors: Audit," *Evening Sun,* 12 Nov. 1991; Department of Fiscal Services, *Sunset Review: State Board of Physician Quality Assurance* (Annapolis: Maryland General Assembly, Oct. 1991), 1–83; Department of Budget and Fiscal Planning, Division of Management Analysis and Audits, *Review of the Board of Physician Quality Assurance* (Annapolis, Md., 1992), 1–60.

149. Maryland Department of Budget and Fiscal Planning, 23.

150. Maryland Department of Fiscal Services, 47; Federation of State Medical Boards, *Exchange* (1992–93), 82. In 1991 the AMA officially endorsed the "Maryland Model" whereby state boards engage the services of professional associations to perform peer review. See Porter, "Ethics and Quality of Care," 91.

151. Maryland Department of Fiscal Services, 50.

152. See VanTuinen et al., *Questionable Doctors*; Wolfe et al., *Questionable Doctors* (1993); "State Medical Boards Discipline Record Number of Doctors in '85," *New York Times,* 9 Nov. 1986; "6,892 Questionable Doctors Identified," *Evening Sun,* 28 June 1990; "Disciplinary Sanctions against Doctors Drop," *Boston Globe,* 22 Apr. 1991; "More Doctors Disciplined under Reforms," *Montgomery Journal,* 15 Apr. 1994; "More Doctors with Violations Keep Their License," *New York Times,* 29 Mar. 1996.

153. See, e.g., Deterling, *Annual Report,* 1; Maryland Department of Fiscal Services, 67.

154. *FSMB News Release,* 24 Apr. 1991.

155. Wolfe et al., *Questionable Doctors* (1996), 11–12. Public Citizen bases its rankings on the number of "serious disciplinary actions" per thousand licensees. "Serious disciplinary actions" include revocations, suspensions, license surrenders, and probations.

156. Interview by author of Bernadette Lane, 11 Apr. 1995.

157. Schattschneider, *Semisovereign People,* 7, 38–40, 118–22.

Chapter 5. The Battle with HMOs

1. Managed-care organizations refer to HMOs, Preferred Provider Organizations (PPOs), Physician Hospital Organizations (PHOs), or any health-care entity that restricts choice of providers, medical options, and physicians' clinical autonomy through treatment protocols. I use the terms *HMO* and *managed-care organization* interchangeably.

2. Taskforce of the Pew Health Professions Commission, *Reforming Health Care Workforce Regulation,* 11.

3. Cf. Mark Cloutier, vice president, Bioethics Consultation Groups, presentation on managed care, annual meeting of the Federation of State Medical Boards, San Diego, Calif., 17 Apr. 1997.

4. Sandra J. Tanenbaum, "Sounding Board: What Physicians Know," *New England Journal of Medicine* 329 (20 May 1993): 1269.

5. Iglehart, "Congress Moves to Bolster Peer Review," 963.

6. Brian McCormick, "Physician Network Broken Up; Antitrust Violations Alleged," *American Medical News,* 15 May 1995, 5–6; Michael Jellinek and Barry Nurcombe, "Two Wrongs Don't Make a Right: Managed Care, Mental Health, and the Marketplace," *JAMA* 270 (Oct. 13, 1993): 1738.

7. Timothy Jost, "Health System Reform," 1508.

8. Andrew Skolnick and Charles Marwick, "Draft of Clinton's Health Reform Plan Draws Cheers, Boos, Polite Applause," *JAMA* 270 (Oct. 6, 1993): 1513–16; Board of Trustees, "Health System Reform Update," in *Proceedings of the House of Delegates* (1993), 189–202.

9. Tanenbaum, "What Physicians Know," 1269; Board of Trustees, "Development of Practice Parameters," in *Proceedings of the House of Delegates* (1989), 80.

10. Jerome Kassirer, "The Use and Abuse of Practice Profiles," *New England Journal of Medicine* 330 (Mar. 3, 1994): 634–35; Linda Prager, "Payers, Providers Open to AMA Profiling Ventures," *American Medical News,* 25 Mar. 1996, 1, 7–8.

11. Jost, "Health System Reform," 1508.

12. Health Security Act, 27 Oct. 1993.

13. James Blumstein, "The Clinton Administration Health Care Reform Plan: Some Preliminary Thoughts," *Journal of Health Politics, Policy and Law* 19 (spring 1994): 204.

14. Congress, House of Representatives, Committee of Ways and Means, *The Health Security Act: Hearing before the Subcommittee on Health* (statement of James R. Winn, M.D.), 103d Cong., 2d session, 1 Feb. 1994, 84, 85.

15. DHEW, *Report on Licensure,* 65–68.

16. Jost, "Health System Reform," 1508; DHEW, *Report on Licensure,* 67.

17. Taskforce of the Pew Health Professions Commission, *Reforming Health Care Workforce Regulation,* 9, 17.

18. Richard D. Lamm, *Critical Challenges: Revitalizing the Health Professions for the Twenty-first Century* (San Francisco: Pew Health Professions Commission, 1995), 12–13.

19. Cf. Abbott, *System of Professions,* 33–58; Ann Martino, executive director, Iowa State Board of Medical Examiners, panel discussion on managed care, annual meeting of the Federation of State Medical Boards, San Diego, Calif., 17 Apr. 1997.

20. Randall R. Bovbjerg, "Promoting Quality and Preventing Malpractice: Assessing the Health Security Act," *Journal of Health Politics, Policy and Law* 19 (spring 1994): 208.

21. Julie Johnsson, "Historic Time: Widespread Managed Care Now Driving Down Prices," *American Medical News,* 2 Jan. 1995, 2, 6–7.

22. Julie Johnsson, "Insurer-HMO Mega-merger," *American Medical News,* 22/29 Apr. 1996, 1.

23. Arnold S. Relman, "Protecting Quality in the Managed Care Era," Platter luncheon and lecture, annual meeting of the Federation of State Medical Boards, San Antonio, Tex., 20 Apr. 1995.

24. Richard M. Lauve, consultant, Louisiana State University, panel discussion on managed care, annual meeting of the Federation of State Medical Boards, San Diego, Calif., 17 Apr. 1997.

25. Israel Weiner, chair, Maryland State Board of Physician Quality Assurance, interview by author, 26 Jan. 1995; Timothy E. Weitz, former legal counsel to the Texas State Board of Medical Examiners, panel discussion on managed care, annual meeting of the Federation of State Medical Boards, San Diego, Calif., 17 Apr. 1997.

26. Leonard Laster, "Managed Care Translates to 'Let the Patient Beware,'" *American Medical News,* 19 Feb. 1996, 18.

27. Jellinek and Nurcombe, "Two Wrongs," 1737–39; Julie Johnsson, "Dad's Protests Lead to Record Fine against California HMO," *American Medical News,* 12 Dec. 1994, 1; Gary F. Krieger, "Examples of New Chaos in Medicine: Six Patient Problems," *American Medical News,* 19 June 1995, 14; Leigh Page, "Law Sought to Ensure Emergency Care," *American Medical News,* 13 May 1996, 4.

28. Nancy W. Dickey, "AMA to Big Managed Care: Ungag Doctors," *American Medical News,* 26 Feb. 1996, 19, 21.

29. Leigh Page, "Market Spawns Doctor-Patient Alliances," *American Medical News,* 13 Nov. 1995, 3, 24; Janice Sommerville, "HMOs Face State Legislative Efforts to Reign Them in," *American Medical News,* 22/29 Apr. 1996, 5–6.

30. According to the *AMA News,* states passed 182 laws affecting managed care in 1997 alone. These laws ran the gamut from HMO report cards and disclosure of financial incentives to mandated benefits. Leigh Page, "States Pass Record Number of Laws on Industry," *American Medical News,* 11 Aug. 1997, 7, 9.

31. Somerville, "HMOs Face State Legislative Efforts," 5. See also Department of State Legislation, *Patient Protection Act (State Version)* (Chicago: American Medical Association, 1994).

32. Page, "Market Spawns Alliances," 24.

33. Janice Somerville, "N.J. Plan Would Let Only Physicians Deny HMO Care," *American Medical News,* 11 Dec. 1995, 4.

34. "State Meetings Embroiled in Managed Care Issues," *American Medical News,* 20 May 1996, 6.

35. Dianne M. Gianelli, "HMO Amends 'Gag Clause'; AMA Calls It 'Good First Step,'" *American Medical News,* 19 Feb. 1996, 4.

36. Rachel Kreier, "Anesthesiologists Sue Aetna: Made Us Skimp Quality," *American Medical News,* 11 Sept. 1995, 4.

37. Janice Somerville, "Decision Gives Doctors New Recourse on HMO Firings," *American Medical News,* 6 May 1996, 6.

38. Julie Johnsson, "New Life for Long-Dormant Law," *American Medical News,* 6 May 1996, 3, 25–26.

39. Board of Trustees, "Practice Parameters," *Proceedings of the House of Delegates* (1991), 88.

40. Linda O. Prager, "Payers, Providers Open to AMA Profiling Ventures."

41. Jerome P. Kassirer, "The Quality of Care and the Quality of Measuring It," *New England Journal of Medicine* 329 (21 Oct. 1993): 1264.

42. Cf. Lynn K. Harvey, *Public Opinion on Health Care Issues* (Chicago: American Medical Association, 1994), 4–9.

43. Council on Ethical and Judicial Affairs, "Ethical Issues on Managed Care," in *Reports of the Council on Ethical and Judicial Affairs of the AMA* (Chicago: American Medical Association, 1994), 278.

44. Ibid., 278–85.

45. Ibid., 280–81.

46. E. Haavi Morreim, "Cost Containment and the Standard of Medical Care," *California Law Review* 75 (1987): 1719–63; Rex O'Neal, "Safe Harbor for Health Care Cost Containment," *Stanford Law Review* 43 (Jan. 1991): 410–21. But cf. Edward B. Hirshfeld, "Should Ethical and Legal Standards for Physicians Be Changed to Accommodate New Models for Rationing Health Care?" *University of Pennsylvania Law Review* 140 (1992): 1842–46.

47. Board of Trustees, "How Cost Containment May Affect the Standard of Care in Medical Malpractice Litigation," in *Proceedings of the House of Delegates* (1991), 121–36.

48. Linda O. Prager, "Gatekeepers on Trial: Primary Care Liability Risks Are Rising with Growth of Managed Care," *American Medical News,* 12 Feb. 1996, 1, 27.

49. Laster, "Managed Care Translates to 'Let the Patient Beware,'" 18.

50. Darling v. Charleston Community Memorial Hospital, 211 N.E. 2d 253 (Ill. 1965).

51. See Hirshfeld, "Ethical and Legal Standards for Physicians," 1816–17, n. 18 and cases cited therein.

52. 239 Cal. Rptr. 810 (Cal. App. 1986).

53. Ibid., 819.

54. Wilson v. Blue Cross of Southern California, 271 Cal. Rptr. 876 (Cal. App. 1990).

55. Fox v. Health Net (Cal. Super. Ct., Dec. 1993); see Gary T. Schwartz, "A National Health Care Program: What Its Effect Would Be on American Tort Law and Malpractice Law," *Cornell Law Review* 79 (1994): 1371–72, n. 136.

56. Prager, "Gatekeepers on Trial," 27.

57. 29 U.S.C.S. secs. 1001–1168.

58. Linda O. Prager, "Aetna Challenges Texas Law Lifting HMO's ERISA Shield," *American Medical News,* 21 July 1997, 1, 25.

59. CIGNA Healthplan of Louisiana, Inc. v. Louisiana ex rel. Ieyoub, CA 5, No. 95-30481, 30 Apr. 1996.

60. Gabriel J. Minc, "ERISA Preemption of Medical Negligence Claims against Managed Care Providers: The Search for an Effective Theory and an Appropriate Remedy," *Journal of Health and Hospital Law* 29, no. 2 (1996): 97–106.

61. 965 F.2d 1321 (5th Cir. 1992), *cert. denied,* 113 S.Ct. 812 (1992).

62. Cuomo v. Travelers (1995) and DeBuono v. NYSA-ILA Medical Clinical Services Fund (1997), as reported by Julie Johnsson, "Supreme Court, Texas Law Strike Blows at ERISA," *American Medical News,* 23/30 June 1997, 6.

63. Prager, "Aetna Challenges Texas Law."

64. Brian McCormick, "When Coverage Decisions Threaten Care: Utilization Review Becomes New Medical Board Concern," *American Medical News,* 20 Feb. 1995, 1, 23; Mark R. Speicher, "Managed Care and the Medical Licensing Community: Is This Ballgame Different?" Presentation at the annual meeting of the Federation of State Medical Boards, Chicago, 11 Apr. 1996.

65. In Maryland, Senate Bill 681 (Discipline of Physician Medical Directors) failed in committee. The legislative packet contained several items of correspondence from medical directors of HMOs opposing the bill.

66. David Yalowitz, M.D., vice president of medical affairs for Prudential Health Care Plan, to the Honorable Ronald A. Guns, 12 Mar. 1996.

67. Plaintiff's Complaint filed in the Superior Court of the State of Arizona, County of Maricopa, John F. Murphy, M.D., and Blue Cross / Blue Shield of Arizona v. Board of Medical Examiners of the State of Arizona, and its acting executive director, Mark R. Speicher (CV94-11501) (hereafter Plaintiff's Complaint), 4.

68. Ibid., 6.

69. Appeal Brief of the Arizona Board of Medical Examiners in *John F. Murphy, M.D. and Blue Cross/Blue Shield of Arizona vs. Board of Medical Examiners of State of Arizona and Mark R. Speicher, Acting Executive Director,* Court of Appeals of Arizona, 1CA-CV95-0321 (hereafter Appeal Brief), 9.

70. Plaintiff's Complaint, 12.

71. Appeal Brief, 20; Maria Kassberg, "Will State Licensing Boards Become Managed Care's Police?" *Managed Care* (Oct. 1995): 48–49.

72. McCormick, "When Coverage Decisions Threaten Care," 23.

73. Speicher, "Managed Care and the Medical Licensing Community."

74. Linda O. Prager, "Arizona Court Upholds Medical Board's Right to Discipline HMO Doctor for UR Decision," *American Medical News,* 11 Aug. 1997, 3, 26.

75. Blue Cross/Blue Shield has indicated that it will file an appeal with the Arizona Supreme Court. Prager, "Arizona Court Upholds Medical Board," 26.

76. Page, "States Pass Record Number of Laws," 9; Prager, "Arizona Court Upholds Medical Board," 26.

77. James Winn, executive vice president, Federation of State Medical Boards, telephone interview by author, 31 May 1996.

78. Linda Oberman Prager, "Mass. Panel Urges Broad Release of Discipline Data," *American Medical News,* 5 June 1995, 4.

79. Speicher, "Managed Care and the Medical Licensing Community."

80. Council on Ethical and Judicial Affairs, "Ethical Issues in Managed Care," 286–88; Linda Oberman Prager, "Doctors Balk at Outsider Oversight, Urge AMA to Seek Role," *American Medical News,* 17 July 1995, 3, 19.

81. Relman, "Protecting Quality in the Managed Care Era."

82. Porter, "Ethics and Quality of Care."

83. Peter E. Dans, M.D., committee member, interview by author, 12 June 1996.

84. Porter, "Ethics and Quality of Care," 90, 92.

85. AMA, Office of General Counsel, *Guidebook for Medical Society Grievance Committees and Disciplinary Committees* (Chicago: American Medical Association, 1991); Edward B. Hirshfeld, AMA, and John M. Peterson, counsel for Chicago Medical Society, to Donald S. Clark, secretary, Federal Trade Commission, 23 Jan. 1992, Special Collections, AMA.

86. Donald S. Clark, secretary, Federal Trade Commission, to Kirk B. Johnson, general counsel, AMA, and John M. Peterson, counsel for Chicago Medical Society, 14 Feb. 1994, at 16, Special Collections, AMA.

87. Linda Oberman, "Board Approach Tries Mediation over Litigation: Massachusetts Tests New Way to Handle Complaints," *American Medical News,* 6 Mar. 1995, 1, 7; Rebecca Arnold Cohen and Dawn Raines, *The Use of Alternative Dispute Resolution by Health Professional Licensing Boards: A Resource Guide* (Washington, D.C.: Citizen Advocacy Center, 1994), 12–14.

88. Cohen and Raines, *Use of Alternative Dispute Resolution,* 19–21.

89. Jost, "Health System Reform," 1509; Taskforce of the Pew Health Professions Commission, *Reforming Health Care Workforce Regulation,* 18–20; Gross, *Foxes and Hen Houses,* 160–85.

90. James S. Todd, "National Practitioner Data Bank: Worthy of Consumer Confidence?" *Federation Bulletin* 80 (winter 1993): 228–29.

91. See Federation of State Medical Boards, *Exchange* (1992–93): 64–65.

92. Fleming, "Massachusetts Physician Profiles," 15–16; *Baltimore Sun,* 5 Nov. 1996.

93. Linda Oberman, "Mass. Society Proposes Controversial Disclosure Rules," *American Medical News,* 13 Mar. 1995, 5.

Chapter 6. State Medical Boards and the New Corporate Order

1. Alexis de Toqueville, *Democracy in America,* ed. Richard D. Heffner (New York: Penguin Books, 1984), 62.

2. See Alfred D. Chandler Jr., *The Visible Hand: The Managerial Revolution in American Business* (Cambridge, Mass.: Harvard University Press, Belknap Press, 1977).

3. Peterson, "Health Care into the Next Century," 292.

4. Ibid.

5. Elizabeth A. McGlynn, "Six Challenges in Measuring the Quality of Health Care," *Health Affairs* 16 (May/June 1997): 12.

6. Emanuel and Emanuel, "Preserving Community in Health Care," 154–55.

7. John Golenski, Ed.D., president, Bioethics Consultation Group, panel discussion on managed care, annual meeting of the Federation of State Medical Boards, San Diego, Calif., 17 Apr. 1997.

8. Morone and Belkin, "The Science Illusion and the Triumph of Medical Capitalism," 3.

9. Cf. Kassirer, "Use and Abuse of Practice Profiles," 634; McGlynn, "Six Challenges," 10.

10. Morone and Belkin, "The Science Illusion and the Triumph of Medical Capitalism," 8.

11. Alain C. Enthoven and Carol B. Vorhaus, "A Vision of Quality in Health Care Delivery," *Health Affairs* 16 (May/June 1997): 46.

12. Ibid., 54–55.

13. Yessian, "Quality of Care Cases."

14. Donald M. Berwick, "Continuous Improvement as an Ideal in Health Care," *New England Journal of Medicine* 320 (5 Jan. 1989): 53–56.

15. Yessian, "Quality of Care Cases."

16. Enthoven and Vorhaus, "Vision of Quality in Health Care Delivery," 48.

17. Ibid., 55; Berwick, "Continuous Improvement," 54.

18. Lawrence L. Weed and Lincoln Weed, "Reengineering Medicine," *Federation Bulletin* 81, no. 3 (1994): 149–83.

19. Pew Health Professions Commission, *Critical Challenges,* 17–20.

20. Yessian, "Quality of Care Cases."

21. Emanuel and Emanuel, "Preserving Community in Health Care," 154–55. See also Linda O. Prager, "What Oversight May Be Overlooking: Mistakes Are Few, but Locus of Monitoring System May Be Outdated," *American Medical News,* 5 June 1995, 1, 22.

22. Schattschneider, *Semisovereign People,* 30.

23. Starr, *Social Transformation of American Medicine,* 14.

24. Haug, "Re-examination of Deprofessionalization," 48–55.

25. Donald Light and Sol Levine, "The Changing Character of the Medical Profession: A Theoretical Overview," *Milbank Quarterly* 66, supp. 2 (1988): 15–19.

26. Cf. Stone, "The Doctor as Businessman," 545.

27. Peterson, "Health Care into the Next Century," 299.

28. Phillip Farell, M.D., Ph.D., dean, University of Wisconsin Medical School, presentation at symposium "Ethical Issues in Managed Care," sponsored by the University of Wisconsin–Madison, 9 May 1996, Policy Paper 97-1.

29. Stone, "The Doctor as Businessman," 550.

30. Yessian, "Quality of Care Issues"; Allen Buchanan, University of Wisconsin School of Business, presentation at symposium "Ethical Issues in Managed

Care," sponsored by the University of Wisconsin–Madison, 11 Apr. 1996, Policy Paper 97-1; Anders, *Health against Wealth,* 244–62.

31. Cf. Jonathan Lurie, *The Chicago Board of Trade, 1859–1905: The Dynamics of Self-regulation* (Urbana: University of Illinois Press, 1979).

32. Corinne Lathrop Gilb, *Hidden Hierarchies: The Professions and Government* (New York: Harper and Row, 1966), 156.

33. William Rock, Dean Medical Center, presentation at symposium "Ethical Issues in Managed Care," sponsored by the University of Wisconsin–Madison, 11 Apr. 1996, Policy Paper 97-1.

34. Michael Millenson, "'Miracle and Wonder': The AMA Embraces Quality Measurement," *Health Affairs* 16 (May/June 1997): 189–93; P. John Seward, "Restoring the Ethical Balance in Health Care," 197.

35. Interview by author of James Winn, M.D., 21 Mar. 1995. See also the remarks of Albert L. Kramer, former Massachusetts judge, who observed that in a competitive marketplace, health facilities will be more tempted to "take care of their mistakes privately, and that's not necessarily in the public interest." Prager, "What Oversight May Be Overlooking," 1.

36. Thomas T. Anton, "New Federalism and Intergovernmental Fiscal Relationships: The Implications for Health Policy," *Journal of Health Politics, Policy and Law* 22 (June 1997): 713–18.

37. Investigative Staff Report, Senate Special Committee on Aging, "Subject; Gaming the Health Care System: Billions of Dollars Lost to Fraud and Abuse Each Year," 7 July 1994.

38. Medicare and Medicaid Patient and Program Protection Act of 1987, 42 U.S.C.A. sec. 1320a-7b (West 1991); Omnibus Reconciliation Act of 1992 (Stark I) and Omnibus Reconciliation Act of 1993 (Stark II), 42 U.S.C.A. sec. 1395nn (West 1991).

39. P.L. 104-191, H.R. 3103.

40. James R. Winn, M.D., executive vice president, Federation of State Medical Boards, and Ellen Riker, MARC Associates, panel presentations on national issues in medical licensure and discipline, annual meeting of the Federation of State Medical Boards, San Diego, Calif., 19 Apr. 1997.

41. William H. Fleming III, M.D., vice president, Board of Directors, Federation of State Medical Boards, panel presentation on health care fraud, annual meeting of the Federation of State Medical Boards, San Diego, Calif., 17 Apr. 1997.

42. Berwick, "Continuous Improvement," 54. Cf. Enthoven and Vorhaus, "A Vision of Quality," 54.

43. Porter, "Ethics and Quality of Care."

44. Andrew and Sauer, "Do Boards of Medicine Really Matter?" 233.

45. Yessian, "State Medical Boards and Quality Assurance," 132–33.

46. Views of Donald Berwick, Institute for Healthcare Quality Improvement, and David Swankin, Citizen Advocacy Center, in Prager, "What Oversight May Be Overlooking," 22.

47. Trish Riley, "The Role of States," 41.

48. Leigh Page, "Clamping Down on Managed Care," *American Medical News,* 11 Aug. 1997, 7–9.

49. Enthoven and Vorhaus, "A Vision of Quality," 55; Peter P. Budetti, "Health Reform for the 21st Century?" *JAMA* 277 (15 Jan. 1997): 197.

50. Bruce Spitz, "Community Control in a World of Regional Delivery Systems," *Journal of Health Politics, Policy and Law* 22 (Aug. 1997): 1042.

51. Francis E. Rourke, "Politics and Professionalism in American Bureaucracy," paper presented at the annual meeting of the American Political Science Association, Chicago, 3–6 Sept. 1992.

Ameringer, Carl F.

State medical boards and the politics of public protection / Carl
F. Ameringer.

p.   cm.

Includes bibliographical references and index.

ISBN 0-8018-5987-5 (alk. paper)

1. Medical care—United States—Quality control.   2. Physicians—
United States—Discipline.   3. Health occupations licensing boards—
United States.   4. Professional standards review organizations
(Medicine)—United States.   I. Title.

[DNLM: 1. Licensure, Medical—United States.   2. Health Policy—
United States.   3. Medicine.   4. Politics—United States.   W 40
AAIA52S 1999]

RA399.A3A47   1999

362.1'0973—dc21

DNLM/DLC

for Library of Congress   98-21738

CIP